slimming slow cooker

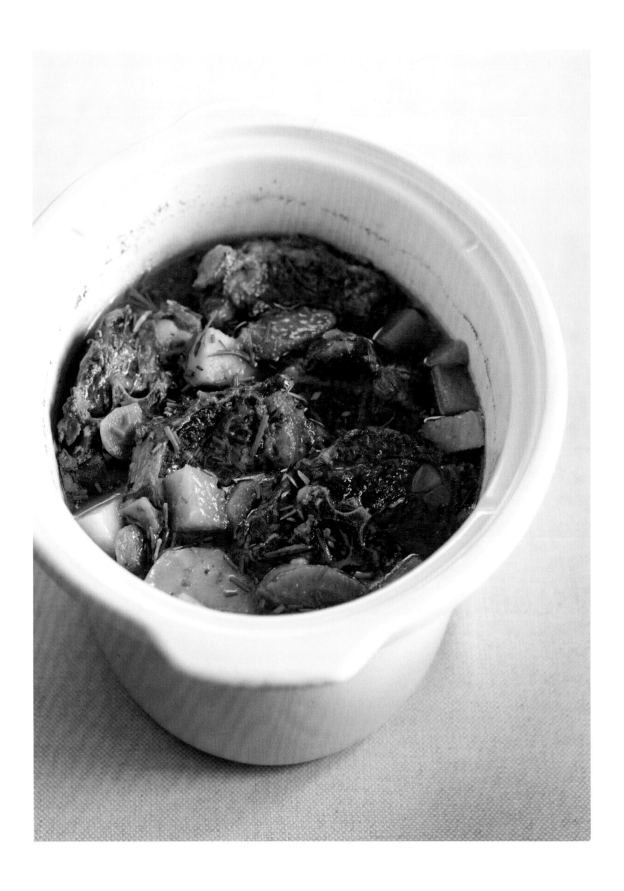

slimming slow cooker

200 RECIPES UNDER 500 CALORIES

hamlyn

First published in Great Britain in 2023
by Hamlyn, a division of Octopus Publishing
Group Ltd, Carmelite House, 50 Victoria
Embankment, London EC4Y 0DZ
www.octopusbooks.co.uk

An Hachette UK Company
www.hachette.co.uk

This material was previously published as
*Hamlyn All Colour Cookery: 200 Light Slow
Cooker Recipes*

Copyright © Octopus Publishing Group Ltd
2023

Distributed in the US by Hachette Book Group
1290 Avenue of the Americas
4th and 5th Floors, New York,
NY 10104

Distributed in Canada by Canadian Manda Group
664 Annette St., Toronto, Ontario,
Canada M6S 2CB

ISBN: 978-0-600-63772-1

A CIP catalogue record for this book is available
from the British Library.

Printed and bound in China

10 9 8 7 6 5 4 3 2 1

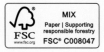

Both metric and imperial measurements
have been given in all recipes. Use one set of
measurements only, and not a mixture of both.
This cookbook uses imperial pints.
1 imperial pint = 2½ US cups

Standard level spoon measurements are used
in all recipes.
1 tablespoon = one 15 ml spoon
1 teaspoon = one 5 ml spoon

Ovens should be preheated to the specified
temperature – if using a fan-assisted oven,
follow the manufacturer's instructions for
adjusting the time and temperature.

Fresh herbs and medium eggs should be used
unless otherwise stated.

The Department of Health advises that eggs
should not be consumed raw. This book
contains some dishes made with raw or lightly
cooked eggs. It is prudent for vulnerable people
such as pregnant and nursing mothers, the
elderly, babies and young children to avoid
uncooked or lightly cooked dishes made with
eggs. Once prepared, these dishes should be
kept refrigerated and used promptly.

This book includes dishes made with nuts
and nut derivatives. It is advisable for those
with known allergic reactions to nuts and nut
derivatives and those who may be potentially
vulnerable to these allergies to avoid dishes
made with nuts and nut oils. It is also prudent
to check the labels of pre-prepared ingredients
for the possible inclusion of nut derivatives.

CONTENTS

INTRODUCTION

about this book

Slimming Slow Cooker is packed with 100 healthy recipes on a variety of topics and cuisines to suit your needs. Every meal included comes with a bonus recipe containing instructions on how to make an exciting variation of the dish, providing you with 200 flavourful recipes in total.

This book is designed to help those people who are trying to lose weight by offering a range of delicious recipes that are low in calories but still high in flavour. The recipes show a calorie count per portion, so you will know exactly what you are eating.

These are recipes for real and delicious food, not ultra-slimming meals, so they will help you maintain a new healthier eating plan for life.

how to use this book

All the recipes in this book are clearly marked with the number of calories (kcal) per serving. There are variations on each recipe at the bottom of the page – note the variation calorie counts as they do vary and can sometimes be more than the original recipe.

The figures assume that you are using low-fat versions of dairy products, so be sure to use skimmed milk and low-fat yogurt. They have also been calculated using lean meat, so make sure you trim meat of all visible fat and remove the skin from chicken breasts.

Use moderate amounts of oil and butter for cooking and low-fat/low-calorie alternatives when you can.

Don't forget to note the number of portions each recipe makes and divide up the food accordingly, so that you know how many calories you are consuming. Be careful about side dishes and accompaniments that will add to calorie content.

Above all, enjoy trying out the new flavours and exciting recipes that this book contains.

SLOW COOKING

If you want to prepare healthy meals but feel you just don't have time, then think again. As little as 15–20 minutes spent early in the day is all that is needed to prepare supper to go into a slow cooker, leaving you free to get on with something else.

Because the food cooks so slowly there is no need to worry about it boiling dry, spilling over or burning on the bottom. Depending on the setting it can be left for 8–10 hours. Slow-cooked food often has much more flavour than dishes prepared in other ways.

When water is added to the pot of a slow cooker it can be used as a bain marie (water bath) to cook baked custards, pâtés or terrines. Alcoholic or fruit juice mixtures can be poured into the pot to make warming party punches or hot toddies. Slow cookers are perfect for steaming puddings, too. Because there is no evaporation you won't have to top up the water or return to find that the pot has boiled dry. The slow cooker pot can also be used to make chocolate or cheese fondues, preserves such as lemon curd or simple chutneys, and you can boil up bones or a chicken carcass for homemade stock.

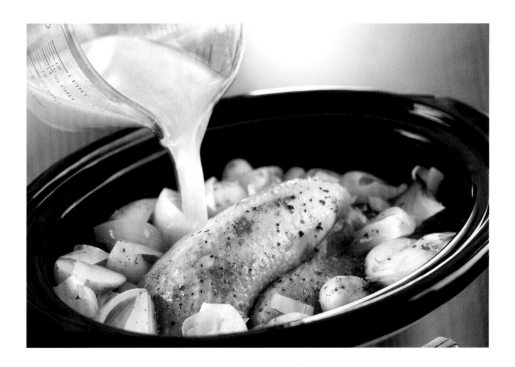

size matters

Unless you have a large family, or like to cook large quantities so that you have enough supper for one meal with extra portions to freeze, you will probably find a slow cooker too big for your everyday needs. Remember that you need to at least half-fill a slow cooker when you are cooking meat, fish or vegetable dishes.

Slow cookers are available in three sizes and are measured in capacity. The size usually printed on the packaging is the working capacity or the maximum space for food:

- For two people, use a mini oval slow cooker with a maximum capacity of 1.5 litres (2½ pints) and a working capacity of 1 litre (1¾ pints).
- For four people, choose a round or more versatile oval cooker with a maximum capacity of 3.5 litres (6 pints) and a working capacity of 2.5 litres (4 pints).
- For six people, you will need a large oval slow cooker with a maximum

capacity of 5 litres (8¾ pints) and a working capacity of 4 litres (7 pints), or an extra large round cooker with a maximum capacity of 6.5 litres (11½ pints) and a working capacity of 4.5 litres (8 pints).

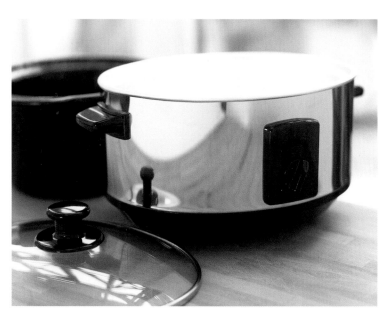

The best and most versatile shape for a slow cooker is an oval, which is ideal for cooking a whole chicken and has ample room for a pudding basin or four individual pudding moulds and yet is capacious enough to make soup for six. Choose one with an indicator light so that you can see at a glance when the slow cooker is turned on.

BEFORE YOU START

It is important to read the manufacturer's handbook before using your slow cooker. Some recommend preheating the slow cooker on High for a minimum of 20 minutes before food is added. Others recommend that it is heated only when filled with food.

how full should the pot be?

A slow cooker pot must only be used with the addition of liquid – ideally it should be no less than half full. Aim for the three-quarter full mark or, if you are making soups, make sure the liquid is no higher than 2.5 cm (1 inch) from the top. Joints of meat should take up no more than two-thirds of the pot. If you are using a pudding basin, ensure there is 1.5 cm (¾ inch) space all the way round or 1 cm (½ inch) at the narrowest point for an oval cooker.

heat settings

All slow cookers have a 'high', 'low' and 'off' setting, and some also have 'medium', 'warm' or 'auto' settings. In general, the 'high' setting will take only half the time of the 'low' setting when you are cooking a diced meat or vegetable casserole. This can be useful if you plan to eat at lunchtime or are delayed in starting the casserole. Both settings will reach just below 100°C (212°F), boiling point, during cooking, but when it is set to 'high' the temperature is reached more quickly. A combination of settings can be useful and is recommended by some manufacturers at the beginning of cooking. (See your manufacturer's handbook for more details.) The following is a general guide to what you should cook at which temperature.

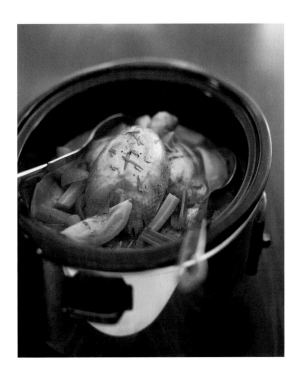

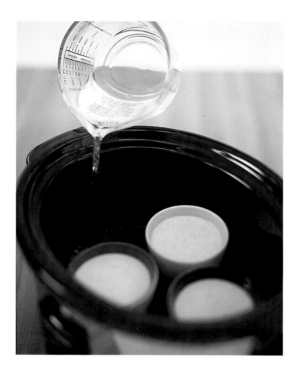

timings

All the recipes in this book have variable timings, which means that they will be tender and ready to eat at the shorter time but can be left without spoiling for an extra hour or two, which is perfect if you get delayed at work or stuck in traffic. Do not change timings or slow settings for fish, whole joints or dairy dishes. If you want to speed up or slow down diced meat or vegetable casseroles, so that the cooking fits around your plans, adjust the heat settings and timings as follows:

LOW	MEDIUM	HIGH
6–8 hours	4–6 hours	3–4 hours
8–10 hours	6–8 hours	5–6 hours
10–12 hours	8–10 hours	7–8 hours

(These timings were taken from the Morphy Richards cooker instruction manual.)

Be aware that as the slow cooker heats up, it forms a water seal just under the lid, but whenever you lift the lid you break the seal. For each time you lift the lid, add 20 minutes to the cooking time. Any pre-cooking is included in the preparation time.

LOW

- Diced meat or vegetable casseroles
- Chops or chicken joints
- Soups
- Egg custard desserts
- Rice dishes
- Fish dishes

HIGH

- Sweet or savoury steamed puddings or sweet dishes that include a raising agent (either self-raising flour or baking powder)
- Pâtés or terrines
- Whole chicken, guinea fowl or pheasant, gammon joint or half a shoulder of lamb.

using your slow cooker for the first time

- Before you start to use the slow cooker, put it on the work surface, somewhere out of the way and make sure that the flex is tucked around the back of the machine and not trailing over the front of the work surface.
- The outside of the slow cooker does get hot, so warn young members of the family.
- Don't forget to wear oven gloves or use tea towels when you are lifting the pot out a heatproof mat on the table or work surface to serve the food.
- Don't put your slow cooker under an eye-level cupboard if the lid has a vent in the top. The steam from the vent could burn someone's arm as they reach into the cupboard.
- Always check that the joint, pudding basin, soufflé dish or individual moulds will fi t into your slow cooker pot before you begin work on a recipe to avoid frustration when you get to a critical point.

preparing food for the slow cooker

MEAT: Cut meat into pieces that are the same size so cooking is even, and fry off meat before adding to the slow cooker. A whole guinea fowl or pheasant, a small gammon joint or half a shoulder of lamb can be cooked in an oval slow cooker pot, but make sure that it does not fill more than the lower two-thirds of the pot. Cover the meat with boiling liquid and cook on high. Check it is cooked either by using a meat thermometer or by inserting a skewer through the thickest part and ensuring that the juices run clear. Add boiling stock or sauce to the slow cooker pot and press the meat beneath the surface before cooking begins.

VEGETABLES: Root vegetables can (surprisingly) take longer to cook than meat. If you are adding vegetables to a meat casserole, make sure you cut them into pieces that are a little smaller than the meat and try to keep all the vegetable chunks the same size so that they cook evenly. Press the vegetables and the meat below the surface of the liquid before cooking begins. When you are making soup, purée it while it is still in the slow cooker pot, using an electric stick blender if you have one.

FISH: Whether you cut the fish into pieces or cook it in a larger piece of about 500 g (1 lb), the slow, gentle cooking will not cause the fish to break up or overcook. Always make sure that the fish is covered by the hot liquid so that it cooks evenly right through to the centre and do not add shellfish until the last 15 minutes of cooking, when the slow cooker should be set to high. Any frozen fish must be thoroughly thawed, rinsed with cold water and drained before use.

PASTA: For best results, cook the pasta separately in a saucepan of boiling water and then mix with the casserole just before serving. Small pasta shapes, such as macaroni or shells, can be added to soups 30—45 minutes before the end of cooking. Pasta can be soaked in boiling water for 10 minutes prior to adding to short-cook recipes.

RICE: Easy-cook rice is preferable for slow cookers because it has been partially cooked during manufacture and some of the starch has been washed off, making it less sticky.

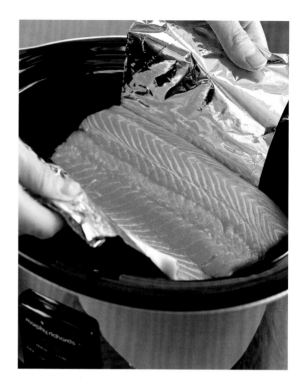

When you are cooking rice, allow a minimum of 250 ml (8 fl oz) water for each 100 g (3½ oz) of easy-cook rice, or up to 500 ml (17 fl oz) for risotto rice.

DRIED PULSES: Make sure that you soak dried pulses in plenty of cold water overnight. Drain them, then put them into a saucepan with fresh water and bring to the boil. Boil rapidly for 10 minutes, skim off any foam, then drain or add with the cooking liquid to the slow cooker. (See recipes for details.)

changing recipes to suit a different model

All the recipes in this book have been tested in a standard-sized slow cooker for four people with a maximum capacity of 3.5 litres (6 pints). You might have a larger 5 litre (8¾ pint) six-portion sized cooker or a smaller 1.5 litre (2½ pint) two-portion cooker.

To adapt the recipes in this book you can simply halve for two portions or add half as much again to the recipe for more portions, keeping the timings the same. All those recipes made in a pudding basin, soufflé dish or individual moulds may also be cooked in a larger slow cooker for the same amount of time.

caring for your slow cooker

If you look after it carefully you may find that your machine lasts for 20 years or more.

Because the heat of a slow cooker is so controllable it is not like a saucepan with burned-on grime to contend with. Once cool, simply lift the slow cooker pot out of the housing, fill the pot with hot, soapy water and leave to soak for a while. Although it is tempting to pop the slow cooker pot and lid into the dishwasher, they do take up a lot of

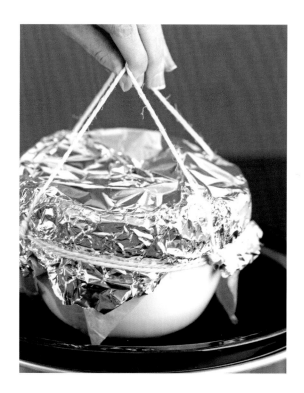

space and not all are dishwasher proof (check your manual).

Allow the machine itself to cool down before cleaning. Turn it off at the controls and pull out the plug. Wipe the inside with a damp cloth, removing any stubborn marks with a little cream cleaner. The outside of the machine and the controls can be wiped with a cloth, then buffed up with a duster or, if it has a chrome-effect finish, sprayed with a little multi-surface cleaner and polished with a duster. Never immerse the machine in water to clean it and if you are storing the slow cooker in a cupboard, make sure it is completely cold before you put it away.

LIGHT BITES

breakfast baked tomatoes

500 g (1 lb) plum tomatoes,
   halved lengthways
leaves from 2–3 thyme sprigs
1 tablespoon balsamic vinegar
salt and pepper
chopped parsley, to garnish
4 slices of wholemeal bread,
   40 g (1½ oz) each, to serve

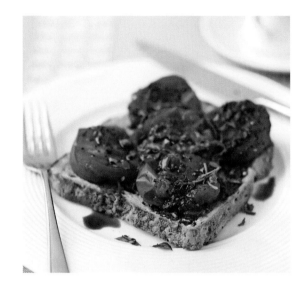

1   Preheat the slow cooker if necessary. Arrange the tomatoes, cut sides up, in the slow cooker pot, packing them in tightly in a single layer. Sprinkle with the thyme, drizzle with the vinegar and season to taste. Cover and cook on Low for 8–10 hours overnight.

for balsamic tomatoes with spaghetti

CALORIES PER SERVING 242

Follow the recipe above to cook the tomatoes, then chop them and mix with the cooking juices. Cook 200 g (7 oz) dried spaghetti according to packet instructions, then drain and toss with the tomatoes. Sprinkle each portion with 1 tablespoon grated Parmesan cheese.

2   Toast the bread the next morning and place on 4 serving plates. Top with the tomatoes and a little of the juice and serve sprinkled with parsley.

brunch poached eggs & haddock

low-calorie cooking oil spray
2 eggs
1 teaspoon chopped chives
2 smoked haddock steaks,
   125 g (4 oz) each
450 ml (¾ pint) boiling water
125 g (4 oz) baby spinach
10 g (½ oz) butter
salt and pepper

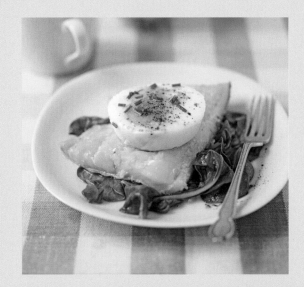

1 Preheat the slow cooker if necessary. Spray the insides of 2 small ovenproof dishes or ramekins with a little low-calorie cooking oil spray, then break an egg into each. Sprinkle with a few chives and season to taste.

2 Place the egg dishes in the centre of the slow cooker pot, then arrange a fish steak on each side. Pour the boiling water over the fish so that the water comes halfway up the sides of the dishes. Cover and cook on High for 1–1¼ hours until the eggs are done to your liking and the fish flakes easily when pressed with a small knife.

for brunch poached eggs with salmon

CALORIES PER SERVING 291

Follow the recipe above, using 2 wild salmon steaks, 100 g (3½ oz) each, instead of the smoked haddock. Arrange 2 sliced tomatoes on the serving plates, top with the cooked salmon and eggs and serve.

3 Rinse the spinach with a little water, drain and place in a microwave-proof dish. Cover and cook in a microwave on full power for 1 minute until just wilted. Divide between 2 serving plates, and top with the fish steaks. Loosen the eggs with a knife and turn out of their dishes on top of the fish. Sprinkle with chopped chives, season with salt and pepper and serve.

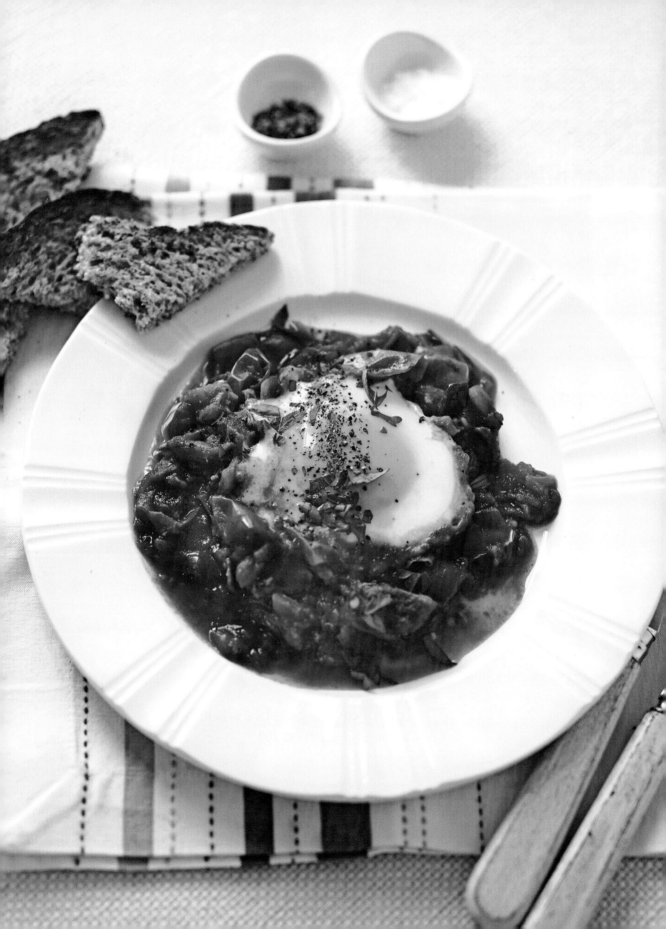

shakshuka

low-calorie cooking oil spray

2 red onions, roughly chopped

75 g (3 oz) chorizo, diced

625 g (1¼ lb) tomatoes, chopped

½ teaspoon dried chilli flakes

1 tablespoon tomato purée

2 teaspoons granular sweetener

2 teaspoons paprika

1 teaspoon dried oregano

4 eggs

salt and pepper

TO SERVE

chopped parsley

4 small slices of wholemeal bread, toasted

1   Preheat the slow cooker if necessary. Spray a large frying pan with a little low-calorie cooking oil spray and place over a medium heat until hot. Add the onion and chorizo and cook for 5 minutes, stirring until the onion has softened.

2   Add the chopped tomatoes, chilli flakes, tomato purée, sweetener, paprika and oregano and season to taste. Transfer the mixture to the slow cooker pot, cover and cook on High for 3–4 hours until the tomatoes have softened and the sauce is thick.

3   Make 4 indents in the tomato mixture with the back of a dessert spoon, then break an egg into each one. Cover again and cook for 15 minutes or until the eggs are set to your liking. Sprinkle with a little chopped parsley, then spoon on to plates and serve with toast.

for mixed vegetable shakshuka

CALORIES PER SERVING 205

Follow the recipe above, omitting the chorizo and using just 1 chopped red onion. Add 1 diced red pepper, 1 large diced courgette, and 2 finely chopped garlic cloves to the frying pan with the onion and continue as above.

baked eggs with toast

25 g (1 oz) butter

4 thin slices of honey roast
ham, 65 g (2½ oz) in total

4 teaspoons spicy tomato
chutney

4 eggs

2 cherry tomatoes, halved

1 spring onion, finely sliced

salt and pepper

4 slices of thinly spread
buttered toast, to serve

1   Preheat the slow cooker if necessary. Use a little of the butter
to grease 4 x 150 ml (¼ pint) ovenproof dishes (checking first
that the dishes fit in your slow cooker pot). Press a slice of
ham into each dish to line the base and sides, leaving a small
overhang of ham above the dish.

2   Place 1 teaspoon of chutney in the base of each dish, then
break an egg on top. Add a cherry tomato half to each,
sprinkle with the spring onion, season to taste, then dot with
the remaining butter. Cover the tops with greased foil and
put in the slow cooker pot.

3   Pour boiling water into the slow cooker pot to come halfway
up the sides of the dishes, cover and cook on High for
40–50 minutes or until the egg whites are set and the yolks
still slightly soft.

4   Remove the foil and gently run a round-bladed knife between
the ham and the edges of the dishes. Turn out and quickly
turn the baked eggs the right way up. Place each on a plate
and serve with the hot buttered toast, cut into fingers.

for eggs benedict

CALORIES PER SERVING 492

Butter 4 dishes as above, then break an egg into each. Season to taste, sprinkle the
eggs with 1 sliced spring onion and dot with 25 g (1 oz) butter. Cover and cook as above.
To serve, grill 8 back bacon rashers until golden. Toast 4 halved English breakfast
muffins, spread with butter, divide the bacon between the lower halves and arrange on
serving plates. Top with the baked eggs and drizzle with 4 tablespoons warmed
ready-made hollandaise sauce. Replace the muffin tops and serve immediately.

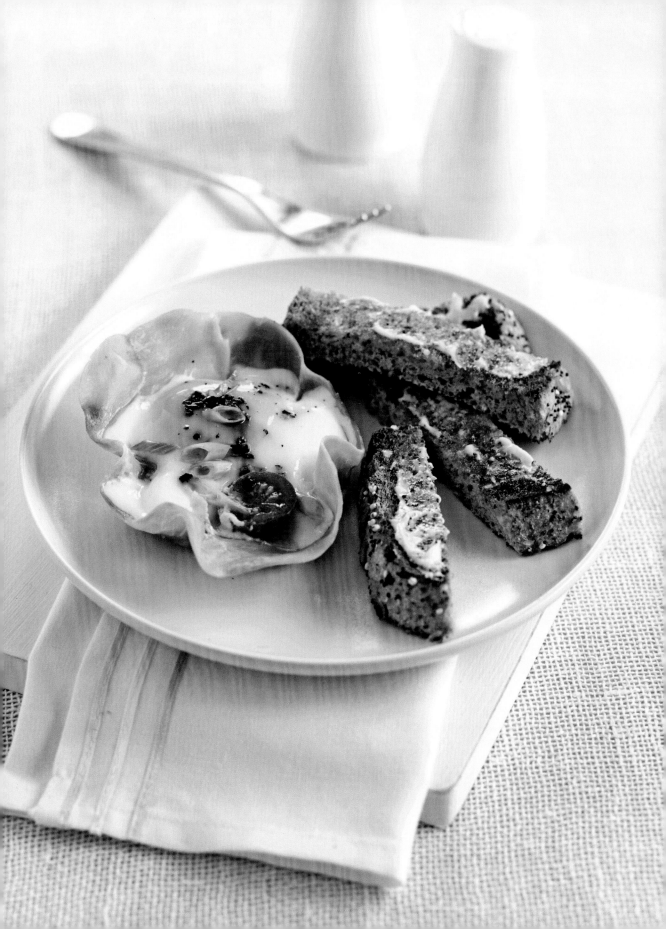

spicy red bean soup

125 g (4 oz) dried red kidney beans, soaked overnight in cold water

2 tablespoons sunflower oil

1 large onion, chopped

1 red pepper, cored, deseeded and diced

1 carrot, diced

1 baking potato 200 g (7 oz), diced

2–3 garlic cloves, chopped (optional)

2 teaspoons Cajun spice mix or ½–1 teaspoon chilli powder

400 g (13 oz) can chopped tomatoes

1 tablespoon brown sugar

1 litre (1¾ pints) hot vegetable stock

50 g (2 oz) okra, sliced

50 g (2 oz) green beans, cut into short lengths

salt and pepper

for paprika & bean soup

CALORIES PER SERVING 252

Follow the recipe above, using 1 teaspoon smoked paprika instead of the Cajun spice and omitting the green vegetables. Purée the soup and add a little boiling water if it is too thick. Ladle into bowls, top each portion with 2 tablespoons soured cream and a few caraway seeds.

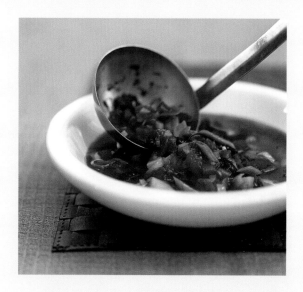

1   Preheat the slow cooker if necessary. Drain and rinse the soaked beans, place in a saucepan, cover with fresh water and bring to the boil. Boil vigorously for 10 minutes, then drain in a sieve.

2   Meanwhile, heat the oil in a large frying pan over a medium heat, add the onion and cook for 5 minutes until softened. Add the red pepper, carrot, potato and garlic (if using) and cook for 2–3 minutes. Stir in the Cajun spice, tomatoes and sugar, season generously and bring to the boil. Transfer the mixture to the slow cooker pot, add the drained beans and hot stock and mix together. Cover and cook on Low for 8–10 hours until the vegetables are tender.

3   Add the green vegetables, cover again and cook for 30 minutes. Ladle the soup into bowls and serve.

chicken noodle broth

1 chicken carcass
1 onion, cut into wedges
2 carrots, sliced
2 celery sticks, sliced
1 bouquet garni
1.2 litres (2 pints) boiling water
75 g (3 oz) vermicelli pasta
4 tablespoons chopped parsley
salt and pepper

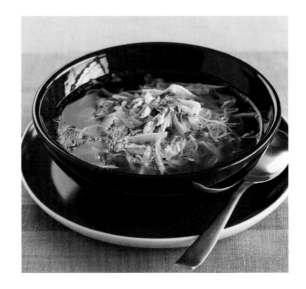

for chicken & minted pea soup

CALORIES PER SERVING 255

Follow the recipe above to make the soup, then strain and pour it back into the slow cooker pot. Add 200 g (7 oz) finely sliced leeks, 375 g (12 oz) frozen peas and a small bunch of mint, cover and cook for a further 30 minutes. Purée the soup in a liquidizer or with a hand-held stick blender, then stir in 150 g (5 oz) mascarpone cheese until melted. Ladle into bowls and sprinkle with extra mint, if liked.

1 Preheat the slow cooker if necessary. Place the chicken carcass in the slow cooker pot, breaking it into 2 pieces if necessary to make it fit. Add the onion, carrots, celery and bouquet garni. Pour over the boiling water and season to taste. Cover and cook on High for 5-7 hours.

2 Strain the soup through a large sieve, then return the liquid to the slow cooker pot. Remove any meat from the carcass and add to the pot. Adjust the seasoning if necessary, add the pasta and cook for a further 20-30 minutes until the pasta is just cooked. Sprinkle with the parsley, ladle into deep bowls and serve.

CALORIES PER SERVING **197** · SERVES **4**
PREPARATION TIME **20 MINUTES** · COOKING TIME **3–5 HOURS**

tomato, pepper & garlic bruschetta

1 large red pepper, quartered, cored and deseeded
500 g (1 lb) plum tomatoes, halved
4 large garlic cloves, unpeeled
leaves from 2–3 thyme sprigs
1 teaspoon granular sweetener
1 tablespoon virgin olive oil
8 slices of French bread, 175 g (6 oz) in total
8 stoned black olives in brine, drained
salt and pepper

1 Preheat the slow cooker if necessary. Arrange the pepper pieces, skin side down, in the base of the slow cooker pot, arrange the tomatoes on top, then tuck the garlic in among them. Scatter the thyme leaves on top, reserving a little to garnish. Sprinkle with the sweetener and drizzle with the oil.

2 Season to taste, cover and cook on High for 3–5 hours until the vegetables are tender but the tomatoes still hold their shape.

3 Lift the vegetables out of the slow cooker pot with a slotted spoon. Peel the skins off the peppers, tomatoes and garlic, then roughly chop the vegetables and toss together. Adjust the seasoning if necessary.

4 Toast the bread on both sides, arrange on a serving plate, then spoon the tomato mixture on top. Arrange the olives and reserved thyme on the bruschetta and serve as a light lunch or starter.

---

for quick tomato & pepper pizzas
CALORIES PER SERVING 237

Follow the recipe above to cook the tomato and pepper mixture, then spoon on to 2 halved and toasted ciabatta rolls. Sprinkle with 50 g (2 oz) grated reduced-fat Cheddar cheese and place under a preheated hot grill to melt the cheese. Serve with salad.

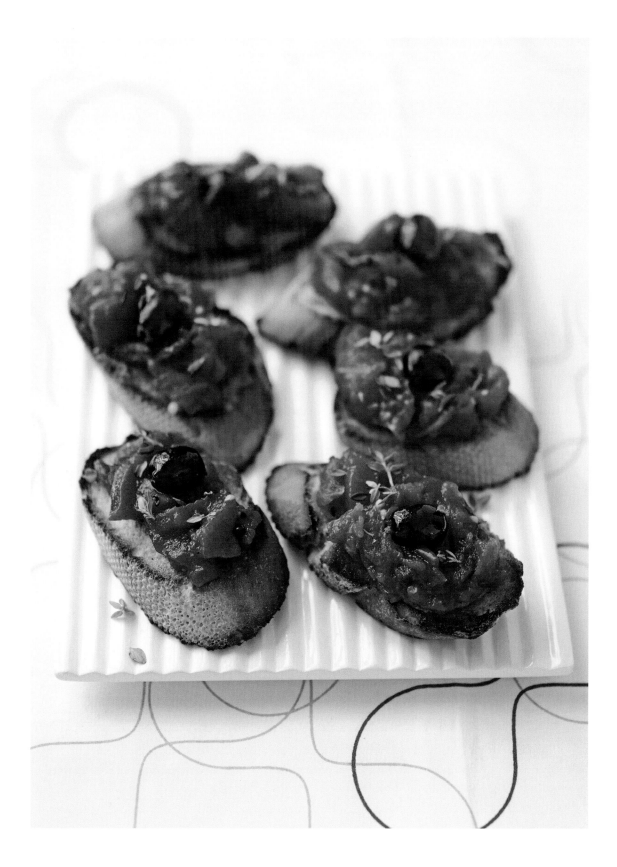

easy cauliflower dal

200 g (7 oz) dried red lentils,
   rinsed in cold water and
   drained
750 ml (1¼ pints) hot water
2 teaspoons medium curry
   powder
½ teaspoon salt
pepper

SPICED CAULIFLOWER
400 g (13 oz) cauliflower, cut
   into small florets
6 tablespoons water
1 onion, thinly sliced
low-calorie cooking oil spray
1 teaspoon cumin seeds,
   roughly crushed
1 teaspoon ground turmeric
1 teaspoon garam masala

1 Preheat the slow cooker if necessary. Place the lentils, hot water, curry powder and salt in the slow cooker pot, then season with pepper. Cover and cook on High for 3-4 hours or until the lentils are soft.

2 Meanwhile, place the cauliflower in a large frying pan with the water, cover and cook over a medium heat for 5 minutes until the cauliflower is almost tender. Drain off any excess water, then add the onion and a little low-calorie cooking oil spray, increase the heat and cook for 2-3 minutes, stirring.

3 Sprinkle the cumin, turmeric and garam masala over the cauliflower and cook, stirring, for 4-5 minutes until the cauliflower is golden brown. Season to taste. Stir the lentil dal, spoon into shallow bowls and top with the spiced cauliflower.

---

for easy aubergine & mushroom dal

CALORIES PER SERVING 201

Follow the recipe above to cook the lentil dal. Spray a large frying pan with a little low-calorie cooking oil spray, add 1 large diced aubergine and 100 g (3½ oz) sliced button mushrooms and cook over a medium heat for 2-3 minutes until beginning to soften. Add a little more low-calorie cooking oil spray, then the cumin, turmeric and garam masala as above and continue to cook until the aubergine is soft. Spoon over the dal and sprinkle with chopped coriander.

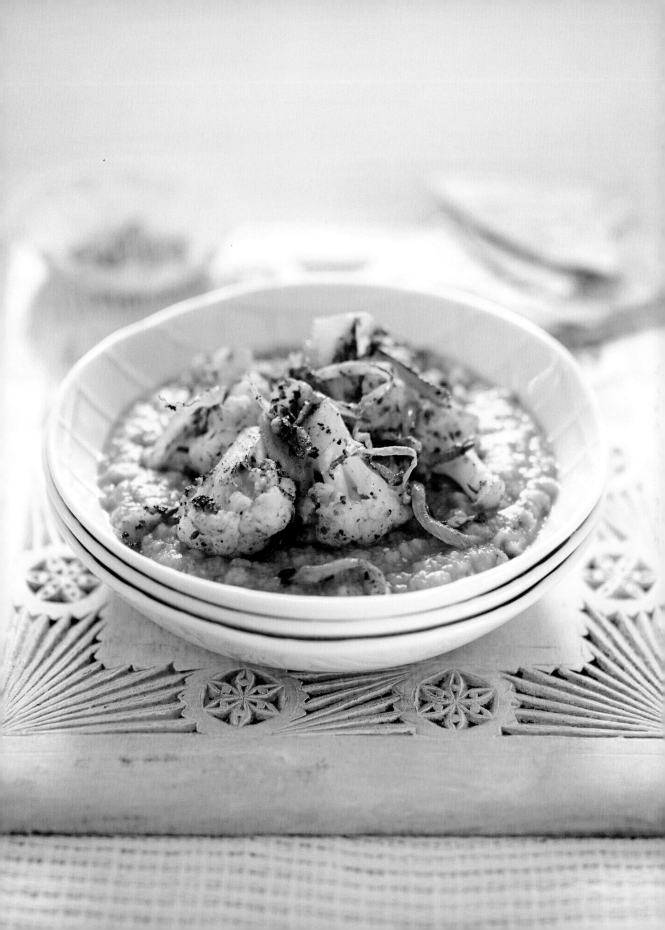

baked peppers with chorizo

2 large red peppers, halved
  lengthways, cored and
  deseeded
2 spring onions, thinly sliced
50 g (2 oz) chorizo, finely diced
200 g (7 oz) cherry tomatoes,
  halved
1–2 garlic cloves, finely
  chopped
small handful of basil, torn, plus
  extra to garnish
4 pinches of smoked hot
  paprika
1 tablespoon balsamic vinegar
salt and pepper

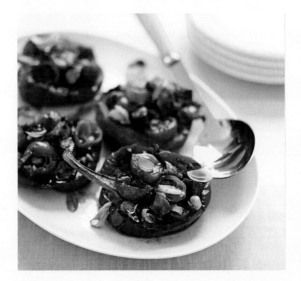

1 Preheat the slow cooker if necessary. Arrange the peppers,
   cut sides up, in a single layer in the base of the slow cooker
   pot. Divide the spring onions and chorizo between the
   peppers, then pack in the cherry tomatoes.

for baked
pepper pizzas

CALORIES PER SERVING 155

Follow the recipe above, omitting
the chorizo and paprika. When
cooked, transfer the peppers to
a shallow ovenproof dish. Tear
150 g (5 oz) mozzarella into small
pieces, sprinkle over the peppers,
then place under a preheated
hot grill for 4–5 minutes until the
cheese is bubbling and golden.
Garnish with extra torn basil and
4 stoned black olives.

2 Sprinkle with the garlic and torn basil, then add a pinch
   of paprika and a drizzle of balsamic vinegar to each one.
   Season to taste, cover and cook on High for 3–4 hours until
   the peppers have softened.

3 Transfer to a platter and sprinkle with extra basil leaves.
   Serve hot or cold as a light lunch with salad.

slow-cooked ratatouille

low-calorie cooking oil spray

1 onion, chopped

1 large aubergine, halved lengthways and sliced

2 garlic cloves, finely chopped

1 red pepper, cored, deseeded and diced

1 orange pepper, cored, deseeded and diced

400 g (13 oz) can chopped tomatoes

150 ml (¼ pint) vegetable stock

1 teaspoon granular sweetener

1 teaspoon dried Mediterranean herbs

2 teaspoons cornflour

500 g (1 lb) courgettes, thickly sliced

200 g (7 oz) cherry tomatoes, halved

salt and pepper

small handful of basil leaves, to garnish

for haricot ratatouille

CALORIES PER SERVING 194

Follow the recipe above, omitting the aubergine and adding a 400 g (13 oz) can of haricot beans, drained, to the frying pan with the stock. Cook as above, then stir in 125 g (4 oz) spinach leaves for the final 15 minutes.

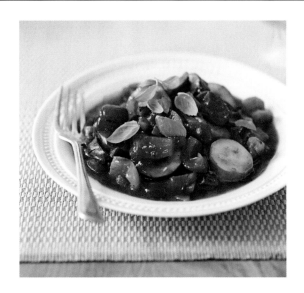

1 Preheat the slow cooker if necessary. Spray a large frying pan with a little low-calorie cooking oil spray and place over a high heat until hot. Add the onion and aubergine and cook for 5 minutes until just beginning to brown.

2 Stir in the garlic, peppers, tomatoes, stock, sweetener and dried herbs, season to taste, then bring to the boil, stirring. Transfer to the slow cooker pot, cover and cook on High for 3–4 hours until the vegetables are tender.

3 Mix the cornflour to a smooth paste with a little cold water and stir into the pot with the courgettes and cherry tomatoes. Cover again and cook for 30–45 minutes until the courgettes are just tender. Garnish with basil and serve.

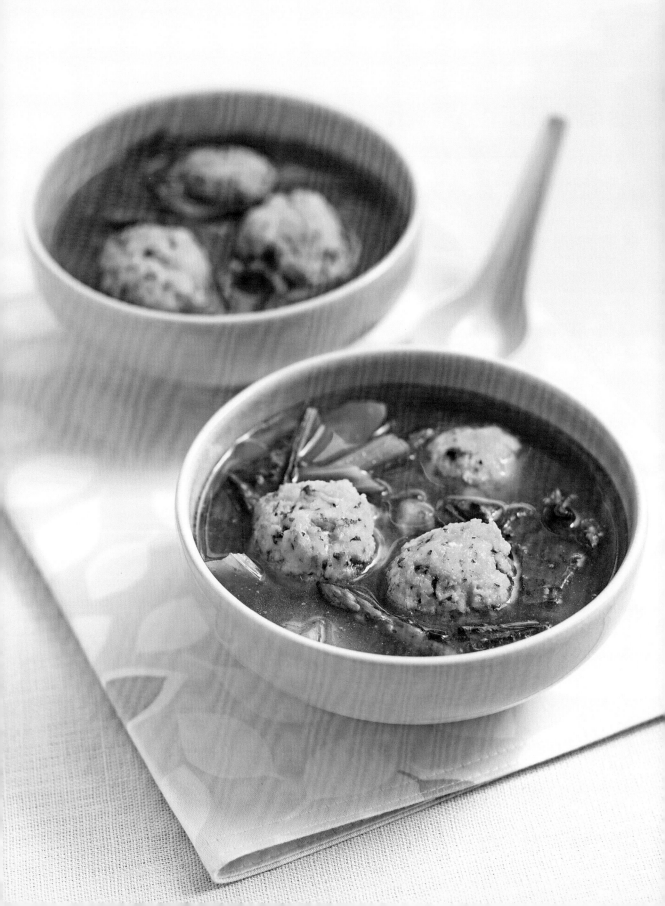

thai-style broth with fish dumplings

900 ml (1½ pints) boiling fish stock

2 teaspoons Thai fish sauce (nam pla)

1 tablespoon Thai red curry paste

1 tablespoon soy sauce

½ bunch of spring onions, sliced

1 carrot, thinly sliced

2 garlic cloves, finely chopped

1 bunch of asparagus, trimmed and stems cut into 4

2 pak choi, thickly sliced

DUMPLINGS

½ bunch of spring onions, sliced

15 g (½ oz) coriander leaves

3.5 cm (1½ inches) fresh root ginger, peeled and sliced

400 g (13 oz) cod, skinned

1 tablespoon cornflour

1 egg white

1 Preheat the slow cooker if necessary. Make the dumplings. Put half of the spring onions into a food processor with the coriander and ginger and chop finely. Add the cod, cornflour and egg white and process until the fish is finely chopped. With wetted hands, shape the mixture into 12 balls.

2 Pour the boiling fish stock into the slow cooker pot, add the fish sauce, curry paste and soy sauce. Add the spring onions, the carrot and garlic and drop in the dumplings. Cover with the lid and cook on Low for 2–3 hours.

3 When almost ready to serve, add the asparagus and pak choi to the broth. Replace the lid and cook on High for 15 minutes or until just tender. Ladle into bowls and serve.

---

for thai-style broth with noodles & prawns

CALORIES PER SERVING 185

Prepare and cook the broth as above, omitting the dumplings, for 2–3 hours. Add the asparagus, pak choi and 200 g (7 oz) frozen large prawns, thoroughly thawed, and cook for 15 minutes on High. Meanwhile, soak 75 g (3 oz) rice noodles in boiling water according to the packet instructions. Drain and add to the bottom of 4 soup bowls. Ladle the broth on top and sprinkle with a little chopped coriander.

roasted vegetable terrine

375 g (12 oz) courgettes, thinly sliced

1 red pepper, cored, deseeded and quartered

1 orange pepper, cored, deseeded and quartered

2 tablespoons olive oil, plus extra for greasing

1 garlic clove, finely chopped

2 eggs

150 ml (¼ pint) milk

25 g (1 oz) Parmesan cheese, grated

3 tablespoons chopped basil

salt and pepper

for romesco sauce to serve as an accompaniment
CALORIES PER SERVING 125

Cook 1 chopped onion in 1 tablespoon olive oil in a frying pan for 5 minutes until softened. Add 2 chopped garlic cloves, 4 skinned and chopped tomatoes, ½ teaspoon paprika and 40 g (1½ oz) finely chopped almonds. Simmer for 10 minutes until thick, season to taste and allow to cool.

1 Preheat the slow cooker if necessary. Line a grill rack with foil and arrange all the vegetables on it in a single layer, with the peppers skin sides up. Drizzle with the oil, sprinkle with the garlic and season with salt and pepper. Grill for 10 minutes or until softened and golden. Transfer the courgette slices to a plate and wrap the peppers in the foil. Leave to stand for 5 minutes to loosen the skins.

2 Oil a 500 g (1 lb) loaf tin and line the base and two long sides with non-stick baking paper, checking first it will fit in the slow cooker pot. Beat together the eggs, milk, Parmesan and basil in a bowl and season to taste. Unwrap the peppers and peel away the skins.

3 Arrange one-third of the courgette slices over the base and sides of the tin. Spoon in a little custard, then add half the peppers in a single layer and a little more custard. Repeat, ending with a layer of courgettes and custard. Cover the top with foil and put in the slow cooker pot.

4 Pour boiling water into the pot to come halfway up the sides of the tin, cover and cook on High for 2–3 hours or until the custard has set. Remove the tin from the slow cooker and leave to cool.

5 Loosen the edges of the terrine with a round-bladed knife, turn out on to a plate and peel off the lining paper. Cut into slices and serve with romesco sauce, if liked.

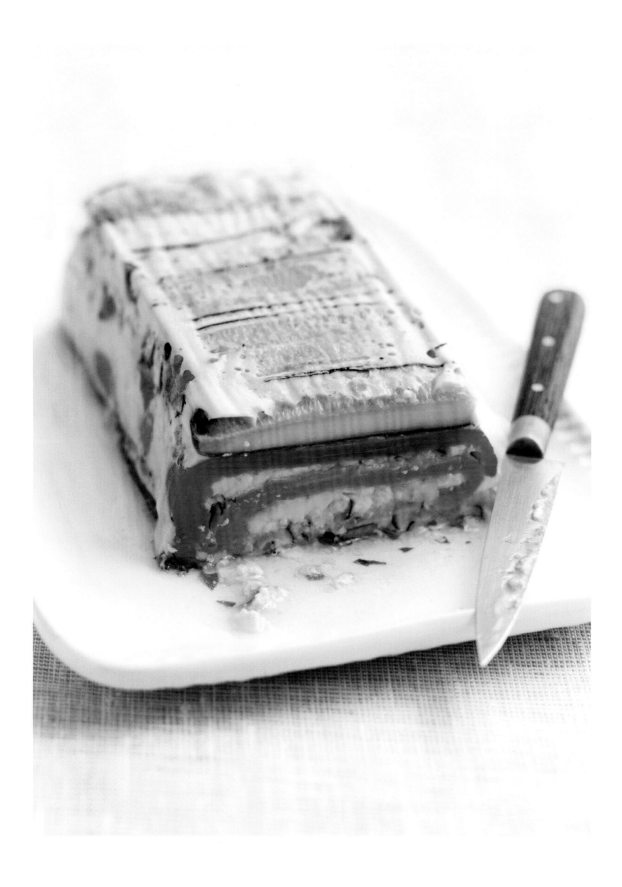

herby stuffed peppers

4 different coloured peppers
100 g (3½ oz) easy-cook brown
  rice
410 g (13½ oz) can chickpeas,
  drained
small bunch of parsley, roughly
  chopped
small bunch of mint, roughly
  chopped
1 onion, finely chopped
2 garlic cloves, finely chopped
½ teaspoon smoked paprika
1 teaspoon ground allspice
600 ml (1 pint) hot vegetable
  stock
salt and pepper

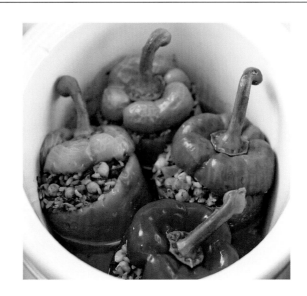

1 Preheat the slow cooker if necessary. Cut the top off each
   pepper, then remove the core and seeds.

2 Mix together the rice, chickpeas, herbs, onion, garlic,
   paprika and allspice with plenty of seasoning. Spoon the
   mixture into the insides of the peppers, then put the
   peppers into the slow cooker pot.

3 Pour the hot stock around the peppers, cover with the lid
   and cook on Low for 4—5 hours or until the rice and peppers
   are tender. Spoon into dishes and serve.

for feta-stuffed peppers

CALORIES PER SERVING 213

Make the recipe as above, but
use 100 g (3½ oz) crumbled feta
cheese, 40 g (1½ oz) sultanas,
a small bunch of chopped basil
and ¼ teaspoon ground allspice
instead of the chopped parsley,
mint, paprika and allspice.

baba ganoush

1 large aubergine, 300 g (10 oz),
    halved lengthways

1 tablespoon olive oil

2 tablespoons 0% fat Greek
    yogurt

3 tablespoons chopped fresh
    coriander leaves

1 large garlic clove, finely
    chopped

juice of ½ lemon

seeds from ¼ pomegranate

salt and pepper

TO SERVE

4 pitta breads

1 red pepper, cored, deseeded
    and cut into batons

½ cucumber, deseeded and
    cut into batons

for grilled steaks with aubergine sauce

CALORIES PER SERVING 294

Make the baba ganoush following the recipe above. Trim the fat from 4 sirloin steaks, 125 g (4 oz) each, and season to taste. Spray with a little low-calorie cooking oil spray and cook on a preheated hot ridged griddle pan for 2–3 minutes, turning once, or until cooked to your liking. Serve the steaks with the baba ganoush and a rocket salad tossed with lemon juice.

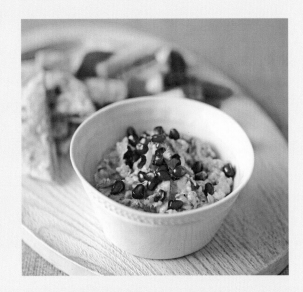

1   Preheat the slow cooker if necessary. Cut criss-cross lines over the cut side of each aubergine half, rub with salt and pepper, then drizzle with the oil. Arrange, cut sides down, in the base of the slow cooker pot, cover and cook on High for 3–4 hours or until the aubergines are soft. Leave to cool.

2   Use a spoon to scoop the flesh out of the aubergine skins and chop it roughly. Place in a mixing bowl with the yogurt, coriander leaves, garlic and lemon juice. Season to taste, spoon into a dish and top with the pomegranate seeds.

3   Warm the pitta breads under a preheated hot grill, then cut into thick strips. Arrange on a serving plate with the pepper and cucumber batons and serve with the baba ganoush.

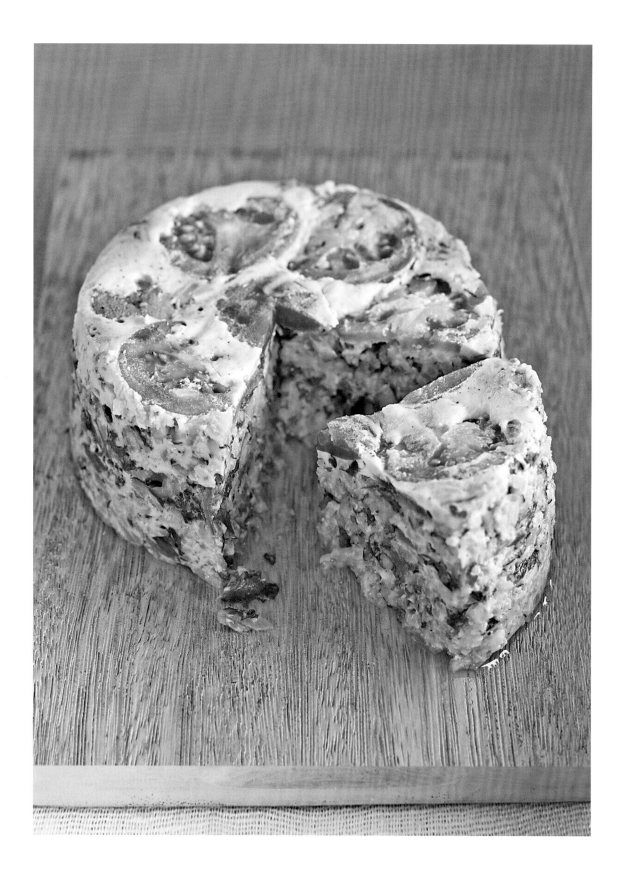

spinach & courgette tian

50 g (2 oz) long-grain rice

1 tablespoon olive oil, plus
extra for greasing

1 tomato, sliced

½ onion, chopped

1 garlic clove, finely chopped

175 g (6 oz) courgettes,
coarsely grated

125 g (4 oz) spinach, thickly
shredded

3 eggs

6 tablespoons milk

pinch of grated nutmeg

4 tablespoons chopped mint

salt and pepper

1 Preheat the slow cooker if necessary. Cook the rice in a saucepan of lightly salted boiling water according to packet instructions until tender.

2 Meanwhile, grease the base and sides of a 14 cm (5½ inch) round ovenproof dish, about 9 cm (3½ inches) deep, with a little oil and line the base with non-stick baking paper. Arrange the tomato slices, overlapping, in the bottom of the dish.

3 Heat the oil in a frying pan over a medium heat, add the onion and cook for 5 minutes until softened. Stir in the garlic, courgette and spinach and cook for 2 minutes or until the spinach has just wilted.

4 Beat together the eggs, milk and nutmeg and season to taste. Drain the rice and stir into the spinach mixture with the egg mixture and mint. Mix well, then spoon into the dish. Cover loosely with greased foil and place in the slow cooker pot.

5 Pour boiling water into the slow cooker pot to come halfway up the sides of the dish, cover and cook on High for 1½–2 hours or until the tian is set in the middle. Remove from the slow cooker, leave to stand for 5 minutes, then remove the foil, loosen the edges and turn out on to a plate. Cut into wedges and serve warm with salad, if liked.

for cheesy spinach & pine nut tian

CALORIES PER SERVING 299

Follow the recipe above, omitting the courgette and stirring 50 g (2 oz) freshly grated Parmesan cheese, a small bunch of chopped basil and 4 tablespoons toasted pine nuts into the mixture instead of the mint.

carrot & cumin soup

1 tablespoon sunflower oil

1 large onion, chopped

625 g (1¼ lb) carrots, thinly
  sliced

1½ teaspoons cumin seeds,
  roughly crushed

1 teaspoon ground turmeric

50 g (2 oz) long-grain rice

1.2 litres (2 pints) vegetable
  stock

salt and pepper

TO SERVE

150 ml (¼ pint) natural yogurt

4 teaspoons mango chutney

4 ready-to-serve poppadums

1 Preheat the slow cooker if necessary. Heat the oil in a large frying pan over a medium heat, add the onion and cook, stirring, for 5 minutes until softened. Stir in the carrots, cumin seeds and turmeric and cook for 2–3 minutes until the onions start to colour.

2 Stir in the rice, then add the stock, season to taste and bring to the boil. Pour into the slow cooker pot, cover and cook on Low for 7–8 hours or until the carrots are tender.

3 Purée the soup in a liquidizer or with a hand-held stick blender until smooth, then adjust the seasoning if necessary and ladle the soup into bowls. Top with spoonfuls of yogurt and a little mango chutney and serve with the poppadums.

---

for spiced parsnip soup

CALORIES PER SERVING 275

Follow the recipe above, replacing the carrots with 625 g (1¼ lb) halved and thinly sliced parsnips. Use 1 teaspoon ground cumin, 1 teaspoon ground coriander and a 3.5 cm (1½ inch) piece of fresh root ginger, finely chopped, instead of the cumin seeds. Continue as above and serve with the yogurt, mango chutney and poppadums.

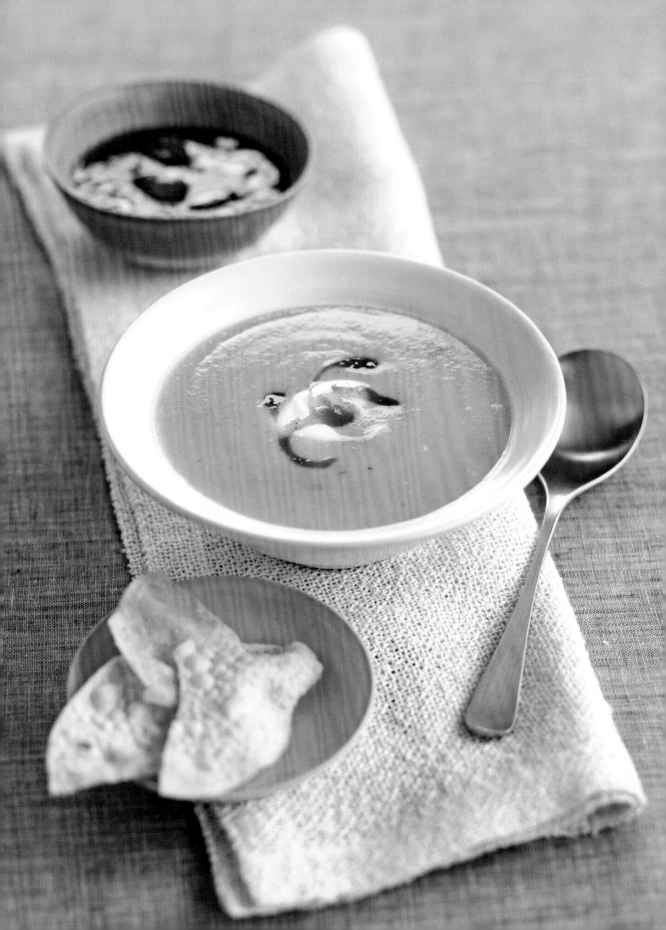

VEGGIE FEASTS

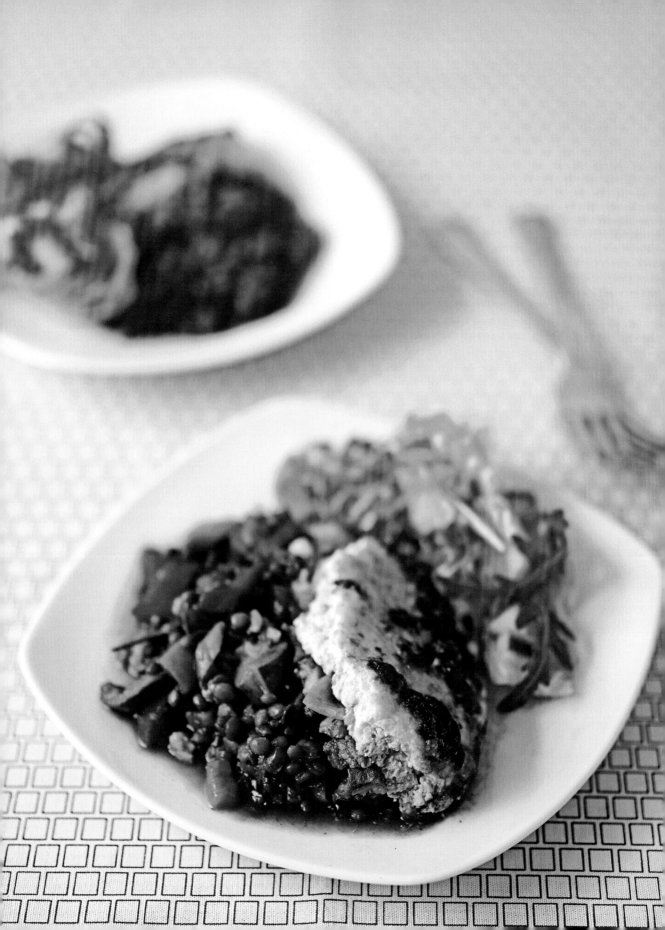

vegetable bake

low-calorie cooking oil spray
1 onion, roughly chopped
1 large aubergine, sliced
2 garlic cloves, finely chopped
1 red pepper, cored, deseeded
  and cut into chunks
1 yellow pepper, cored,
  deseeded and cut into chunks
2 large courgettes, thickly sliced
500 g (1 lb) passata
150 ml (¼ pint) vegetable stock
75 g (3 oz) dried Puy lentils
leaves from 3 rosemary sprigs,
  chopped
1 teaspoon granular sweetener
salt and pepper

TOPPING
250 ml (8 fl oz) 0% fat Greek
  yogurt
3 eggs
25 g (1 oz) grated Parmesan

1 Preheat the slow cooker if necessary. Spray a large frying pan with a little low-calorie cooking oil spray and place over a high heat until hot. Add the onion and aubergine and fry for 4–5 minutes, stirring until just beginning to brown. Add the garlic, peppers and courgettes and cook for 2 minutes more, then add the passata, stock and lentils.

2 Add the rosemary and sweetener and season to taste. Bring to a boil, stirring, then transfer to the slow cooker pot. Cover and cook on Low for 6–8 hours until the lentils are tender.

3 Mix the yogurt, eggs and a little pepper together in a bowl until smooth. Stir the vegetable mixture, then smooth the surface with the back of a spoon. Pour the yogurt mixture over the top in an even layer and sprinkle with the Parmesan. Cover and continue cooking for 45 minutes–1¼ hours until the custard has set.

4 Place the slow cooker pot under a preheated hot grill for 4–5 minutes until the top is golden, then serve with a green salad, if liked.

for penne with vegetables
CALORIES PER SERVING 399

Make and cook the vegetable and lentil mixture as above. Cook 90 g (3¼ oz) dried wholewheat penne pasta in a saucepan of lightly salted boiling water according to packet instructions. Drain and stir into the cooked vegetables, spoon into shallow dishes and sprinkle with 25 g (1 oz) grated Parmesan cheese.

spiced date & chickpea pilaf

1 tablespoon olive oil

1 onion, chopped

1–2 garlic cloves, finely
chopped

4 cm (1½ inch) piece of fresh
root ginger, finely chopped

1 teaspoon ground turmeric

1 teaspoon ground cumin, plus
extra to garnish

1 teaspoon ground coriander

200 g (7 oz) easy-cook brown
rice, boiled

400 g (13 oz) can chickpeas,
drained

75 g (3 oz) pitted dates,
chopped

1 litre (1¾ pints) vegetable stock

salt and pepper

TO SERVE

1 tablespoon olive oil

1 onion, thinly sliced

150 ml (¼ pint) 0% fat
Greek yogurt

small handful of chopped fresh
coriander

1 Preheat the slow cooker if necessary. Heat the oil in a large frying pan over a medium heat, add the onion and cook for 5 minutes until softened. Stir in the garlic, ginger and ground spices and cook for 1 minute.

2 Add the rice, chickpeas, dates and stock, season to taste and bring to the boil, stirring. Pour into the slow cooker pot, cover and cook on Low for 3–4 hours until the rice is tender and nearly all the stock has been absorbed.

3 Meanwhile, heat the remaining oil in a frying pan over a medium heat, add the sliced onion and cook, stirring, until crisp and golden.

4 Stir the pilaf, spoon into bowls and top each portion with a spoonful of yogurt, a little extra cumin, some crispy onions and a little chopped coriander.

---

for almond & 'fake chicken' pilaf

CALORIES PER SERVING 459

Follow the recipe above, adding 300 g (10 oz) mycoprotein vegetarian chicken pieces to the frying pan with the chopped onion. Continue as above, omitting the dates. To serve, top with 25 g (1 oz) toasted flaked almonds, the Greek yogurt and a little chopped mint instead of the crispy onions and coriander.

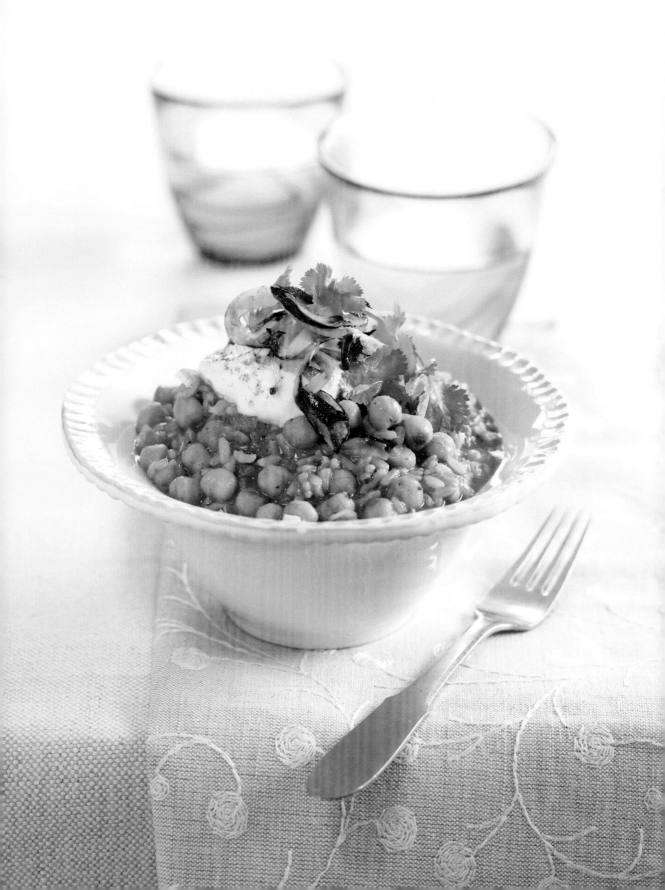

chilli, mushroom & tomato pasta

1 tablespoon olive oil

1 red onion, roughly chopped

2 garlic cloves, finely chopped

1 teaspoon paprika

½ teaspoon dried chilli flakes

1 teaspoon dried
   Mediterranean herbs

400 g (13 oz) passata

2 teaspoons granular
   sweetener

300 g (10 oz) small button
   mushrooms

300 g (10 oz) cherry tomatoes

salt and pepper

TO SERVE

200 g (7 oz) dried penne pasta

large pinch of dried chilli

flakes (optional) handful of
   rocket leaves

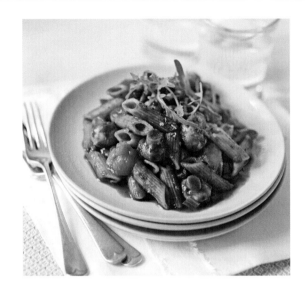

1 Preheat the slow cooker if necessary. Heat the oil a large frying pan over a medium heat until hot, add the onion and cook for 4–5 minutes, stirring until just beginning to soften. Add the garlic, paprika and chilli flakes, then the dried herbs, passata and sweetener. Season to taste and bring to the boil.

2 Place the mushrooms and cherry tomatoes in the slow cooker pot, pour over the hot passata mixture and stir well. Cover and cook on Low for 7–8 hours.

3 Cook the pasta in a saucepan of lightly salted boiling water according to packet instructions until tender. Drain and stir into the ragu, then spoon into shallow bowls and sprinkle with a few extra dried chilli flakes, if liked, and top with the rocket. Serve immediately.

for courgette & tomato arrabiata

CALORIES PER SERVING 307

Follow the recipe above, using 200 g (7 oz) diced courgette and 1 cored, deseeded and diced red pepper instead of the mushrooms.

beetroot & caraway risotto

200 g (7 oz) long-grain brown
  rice
300 g (10 oz) beetroot, diced
1 red onion, finely chopped
2 garlic cloves, finely chopped
1 teaspoon caraway seeds
2 teaspoons tomato purée
1.2 litres (2 pints) hot
  vegetable stock
salt and pepper

TO SERVE
4 tablespoons Greek yogurt
125 g (4 oz) smoked salmon
  slices
handful of rocket leaves

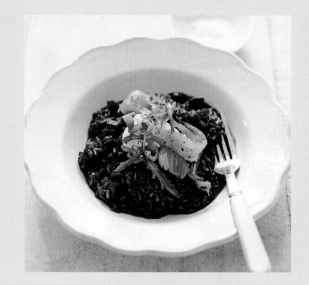

1   Preheat the slow cooker if necessary. Place the rice in a sieve, rinse well under cold running water and drain well.

2   Place the beetroot, onion and garlic in the slow cooker pot, add the drained rice, caraway seeds and tomato purée, then stir in the hot stock and season generously. Cover and cook on Low for 5–6 hours until the rice and beetroot are tender.

3   Stir the risotto, spoon on to plates and top each portion with a spoonful of yogurt, some smoked salmon and a few rocket leaves. Serve immediately.

for pumpkin & sage risotto
CALORIES PER SERVING 354

Place 300 g (10 oz) diced pumpkin in the slow cooker pot with 1 finely chopped white onion and 2 chopped garlic cloves. Mix in 250 g (8 oz) rinsed brown rice and flavour with 2 sage sprigs, 1 teaspoon paprika and 2 teaspoons tomato purée. Add 1.2 litres (2 pints) hot vegetable stock, season and cook as above. Serve sprinkled with 75 g (3 oz) finely grated Parmesan cheese.

aubergine parmigiana

1 tablespoon olive oil

1 onion, chopped

2 garlic cloves, finely chopped

400 g (13 oz) tomatoes, diced

400 g (13 oz) can chopped
tomatoes

small handful of basil, torn,
plus extra to garnish

2 teaspoons granular
sweetener

2 teaspoons cornflour

2 large aubergines, sliced

75 g (3 oz) mature Cheddar
cheese, grated

salt and pepper

2 tablespoons finely grated
Parmesan cheese, to garnish

1 Preheat the slow cooker if necessary. Heat the oil in a large frying pan over a medium heat, add the onion and cook for 4–5 minutes until just beginning to soften. Add the garlic, fresh tomatoes, canned tomatoes, basil and sweetener. Mix the cornflour to a smooth paste with a little cold water and stir into the sauce. Season to taste and bring to the boil, stirring.

2 Spoon a little of the tomato sauce over the base of the slow cooker pot and arrange one-third of the aubergine slices, overlapping, on top. Spoon over a thin layer of the sauce and sprinkle with a little grated Cheddar. Repeat to make 3 aubergine layers, finishing with a generous layer of sauce and grated Cheddar.

3 Cover and cook on High for 4–5 hours until the aubergines are soft. Sprinkle with the Parmesan and extra basil and serve.

for mushroom parmigiana

CALORIES PER SERVING 235

Follow the recipe above to make the tomato sauce, then layer in the slow cooker pot with 8 large flat field mushrooms, in 2 layers, and the Cheddar. Cook and serve as above.

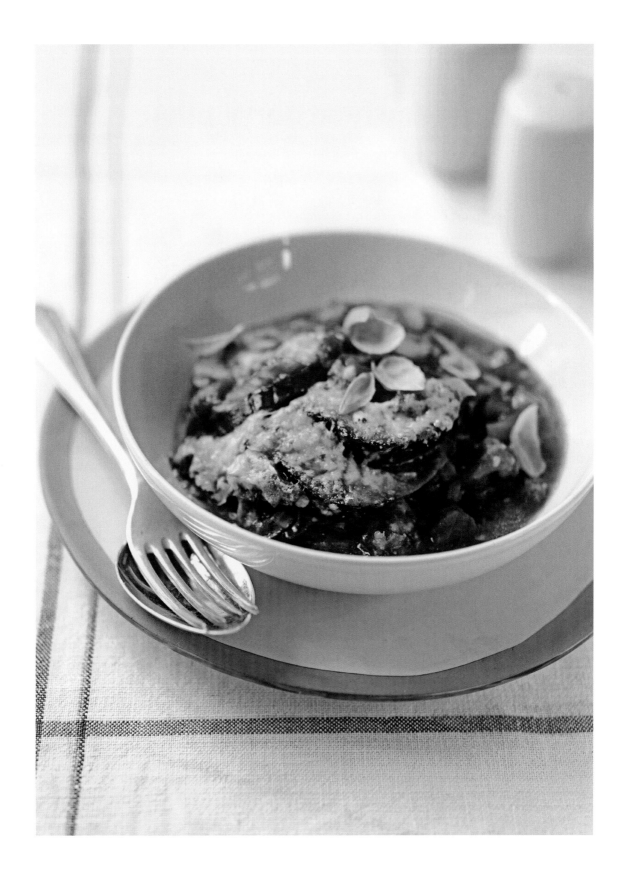

mushroom & wheatberry pilau

1 tablespoon olive oil

1 onion, thinly sliced

2 garlic cloves, finely chopped

325 ml (11 fl oz) brown ale

450 ml (¾ pint) vegetable
  stock

3 sage sprigs

¼ teaspoon grated nutmeg

5 cm (2 inch) cinnamon stick

1 tablespoon sun-dried tomato
  paste

200 g (7 oz) wheatberries

250 g (8 oz) chestnut
  mushrooms, halved

250 g (8 oz) large closed-cap
  mushrooms, quartered

salt and pepper

15 g (½ oz) parsley, roughly
  chopped, to garnish

1 Preheat the slow cooker if necessary. Heat the oil in a large frying pan over a medium heat until hot. Add the onion and fry for 4–5 minutes, stirring until just beginning to soften. Add the garlic, brown ale, stock, sage, nutmeg and cinnamon. Stir in the tomato paste and season well, then bring to the boil.

2 Place the wheatberries and mushrooms in the slow cooker pot. Pour over the hot ale mixture, then cover and cook on High for 3½–4 hours until the wheatberries are tender and nearly all the liquid has been absorbed. Stir well, then sprinkle with the parsley. Spoon into shallow bowls to serve.

for red pepper wheatberry pilau

CALORIES PER SERVING 363

Fry 1 sliced red onion in the oil as above, then add 2 finely chopped garlic cloves and 2 cored, deseeded and sliced red peppers. Stir in 200 ml (7 fl oz) red wine, 600 ml (1 pint) vegetable stock, a small handful of basil leaves and 1 tablespoon sun-dried tomato paste. Season to taste and bring to the boil, then pour over the wheatberries in the slow cooker pot and cook as above.

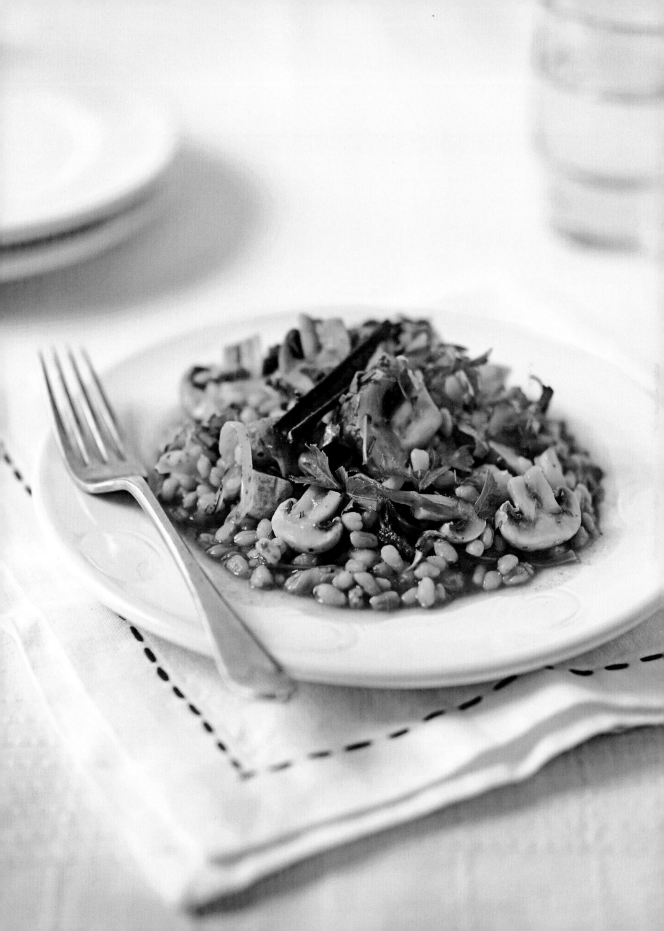

hot quinoa & pepper salad

3 peppers, cored, deseeded,
and cut into chunks
2 celery sticks, sliced
2 courgettes, halved
lengthways and thickly sliced
250 g (8 oz) plum tomatoes,
roughly chopped
2 garlic cloves, finely chopped
125 g (4 oz) quinoa and bulgur
wheat grain mix
4 tablespoons red wine
300 ml (½ pint) hot vegetable
stock
1 tablespoon tomato purée
1 teaspoon granular sweetener
15 g (½ oz) basil leaves, roughly
torn
salt and pepper

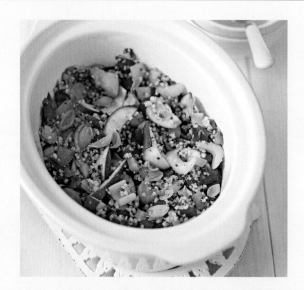

1 Preheat the slow cooker if necessary. Place the peppers,
celery, courgettes and tomatoes in the slow cooker pot and
sprinkle over the garlic and grain mix.

2 Mix the red wine with the stock, tomato purée and
sweetener, season to taste and pour into the slow cooker
pot. Stir the ingredients together, then cover and cook on
High for 3-4 hours until the vegetables have softened and
the grains have absorbed the liquid.

for hot quinoa & tofu salad

CALORIES PER SERVING 199

Follow the recipe above to make
the quinoa salad and divide
between 4 bowls. Omit the basil
and divide 100 g (3½ oz) mixed
spinach, watercress and rocket
leaves and 300 g (10 oz) tofu
between the bowls.

3 Stir the salad, then divide between 4 shallow bowls and
serve topped with the torn basil leaves.

smoky sweet potato 'chilli'

1–2 small dried smoked chipotle
   chillies
4 tablespoons boiling water
low-calorie cooking oil spray
1 onion, chopped
2 garlic cloves, finely chopped
1 teaspoon ground cumin
1 teaspoon paprika
2 x 400 g (13 oz) cans chopped
   tomatoes
400 g (13 oz) can red kidney
   beans, rinsed and drained
350 g (11½ oz) mycoprotein
   mince
300 g (10 oz) sweet potato, cut
   into 2.5 cm (1 inch) cubes
salt and pepper

SALSA
½ red onion, finely chopped
3 tablespoons chopped fresh
   coriander
2 tomatoes, halved, deseeded
   and diced

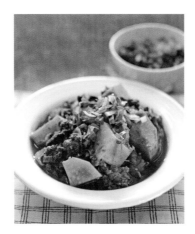

1   Preheat the slow cooker
    if necessary. Place the
    dried chillies in a small
    bowl, pour over the boiling
    water and leave to stand
    for 10 minutes.

2   Spray a large frying pan
    with a little low-calorie
    cooking oil spray and
    place over a medium heat
    until hot. Add the onion,
    fry for 4–5 minutes until
    softened, then add the
    garlic, cumin and paprika.
    Stir in the tomatoes and
    kidney beans, then add
    the mycoprotein and
    sweet potato. Season
    to taste.

3   Finely chop the chillies,
    then stir into the
    mycoprotein mixture with
    the soaking water. Bring
    to the boil, stirring, then
    transfer to the slow cooker
    pot. Cover and cook on
    Low for 7–8 hours until the
    sweet potato is tender.
    Mix the salsa ingredients
    together, then sprinkle
    over the chilli to serve.

for sweet potato & lentil curry

CALORIES PER SERVING 299

Follow the recipe above,
omitting the chipotle chillies.
Add 1 teaspoon ground turmeric,
1 teaspoon garam masala and
½ teaspoon dried chilli flakes
with the cumin and paprika,
and a 400 g (13 oz) can lentils,
drained, when adding the
mycoprotein mince. Cook as
above, then add 100 g (3½ oz)
frozen peas and 4 tablespoons
chopped fresh coriander, cover
again and cook on High for
15 minutes.

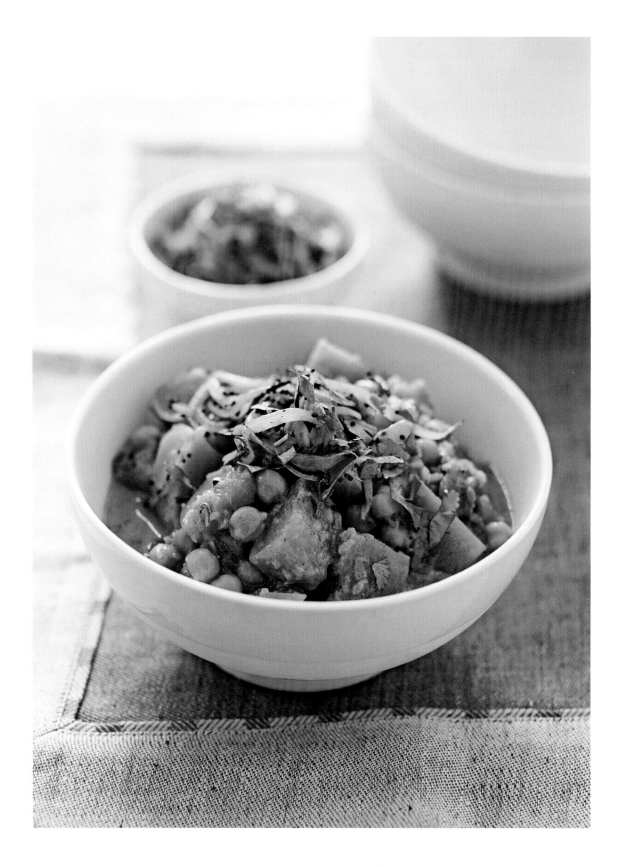

coconut, pumpkin & chickpea curry

2 onions

2 garlic cloves, halved

4 cm (1½ inch) piece of fresh
   root ginger, sliced

1 red chilli, quartered and
   deseeded

low-calorie cooking oil spray

1½ tablespoons medium curry
   powder

1 teaspoon fennel seeds,
   roughly crushed

200 ml (7 fl oz) full-fat
   coconut milk

300 ml (½ pint) vegetable
   stock

2 teaspoons granular
   sweetener

650 g (1 lb 5 oz) peeled
   pumpkin, cut into 4 cm
   (1½ inch) chunks

400 g (13 oz) can chickpeas,
   drained

1 teaspoon black mustard
   seeds

15 g (½ oz) fresh coriander,
   roughly torn

juice of 1 lime

salt and pepper

1 Preheat the slow cooker if necessary. Quarter 1 of the
onions and place with the onion, garlic, ginger and chilli
in a food processor and blitz until very finely chopped.
Alternatively, chop the ingredients finely with a knife.
Spray a large frying pan with a little low-calorie cooking oil
spray and place over a high heat until hot. Add the onion
paste and cook for 2 minutes, then stir in the curry powder
and fennel seeds.

2 Add the coconut milk, stock and sweetener, then season
to taste. Bring to the boil, stirring. Place the pumpkin and
chickpeas in the slow cooker pot and pour the coconut
mixture on top. Cover and cook on Low for 6–8 hours until
the pumpkin is tender.

3 Make a crispy onion topping by slicing the remaining onion.
Heat a little low-calorie cooking oil spray in a clean frying
pan and cook the onion over a medium heat for 5 minutes
until softened. Stir in the mustard seeds and cook for a few
minutes more until the onion is golden and crispy. Stir the
coriander and lime juice into the curry, spoon into bowls and
served topped with the crispy onions.

---

for creamy coconut, aubergine & chickpea curry

CALORIES PER SERVING 246

Follow the recipe above, using 625 g (1¼ lb) aubergines, trimmed
and diced, instead of the pumpkin.

---

vegetable sausages with onion gravy

low-calorie cooking oil spray

2 x 240 g (7½ oz) packets of
  soya sausages

300 g (10 oz) onions, thinly
  sliced

2 teaspoons dark muscovado
  sugar

350 ml (12 fl oz) vegetable
  stock

1 tablespoon tomato purée

2 teaspoons wholegrain
  mustard

2 teaspoons cornflour

salt and pepper

675 g (1 lb 6 oz) celeriac, cubed
  just before cooking

chopped parsley, to garnish
  (optional)

TO SERVE

360 g (11¾ oz) fine green
  beans, steamed

1   Preheat the slow cooker if necessary. Spray a large frying pan with a little low-calorie cooking oil spray and place over a high heat until hot. Add the sausages and cook for 2–3 minutes until browned all over. Transfer to the slow cooker pot in a single layer.

2   Add a little extra low-calorie cooking oil spray to the frying pan, add the onions and cook over a medium heat for 5 minutes until just beginning to soften. Add the sugar and continue to cook for 5 minutes until deep brown, being careful not to burn the onions.

3   Stir in the stock, tomato purée and mustard. Mix the cornflour to a smooth paste with a little cold water and stir into the pan. Season to taste and bring to the boil, stirring. Pour over the sausages, cover and cook on High for 4–5 hours until the sausages are cooked through.

4   Cook the celeriac in a saucepan of lightly salted boiling water for 15–20 minutes until tender. Drain and mash the celeriac with 3–4 tablespoons of the cooking water and season to taste. Divide the mash between 4 serving plates and top with the sausages and onion gravy. Sprinkle with a little chopped parsley, if liked, and serve with the steamed green beans.

---

for vegetable sausages with sweet potato

CALORIES PER SERVING 424

Follow the recipe above to make the onion gravy and vegetable sausages. Instead of the celeriac mash, cut 360 g (12 ½ oz) sweet potatoes into chunks. Steam or boil until tender, then mash with 2 tablespoons crème fraîche and a good grinding of nutmeg. Season with salt and pepper. Serve with parsley and green beans, as above.

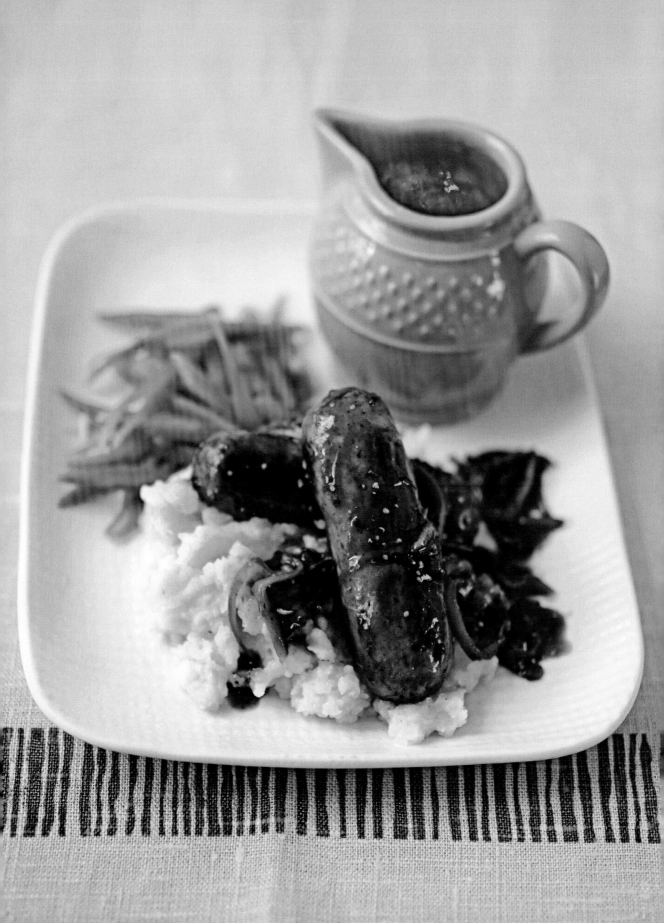

lentil tagine with pomegranate

1 tablespoon olive oil

1 onion, chopped

5 cm (2 inch) piece of fresh root
  ginger, finely chopped

3 garlic cloves, finely chopped

2 teaspoons cumin seeds, crushed

1 teaspoon coriander seeds, crushed

200 g (7 oz) dried Puy lentils

2 celery sticks, sliced

250 g (8 oz) cherry tomatoes, halved

450 ml (¾ pint) hot vegetable stock

juice of 1 lemon

15 g (½ oz) flat-leaf parsley,
  roughly chopped

15 g (½ oz) mint, roughly chopped

salt and pepper

TO SERVE

125 ml (4 fl oz) 0% fat Greek yogurt

1 tablespoon harissa

seeds from ½ pomegranate

for chickpea & lentil tagine

CALORIES PER SERVING 256

Follow the recipe above, adding
½ teaspoon chilli powder with the
other spices and using 100 g (3½ oz)
Puy lentils and a 400 g (13 oz) can
of chickpeas, drained, instead of
200 g (7 oz) lentils. Omit the mint
and pomegranate, but stir in 25 g (1
oz) parsley and serve topped with
the yogurt and harissa.

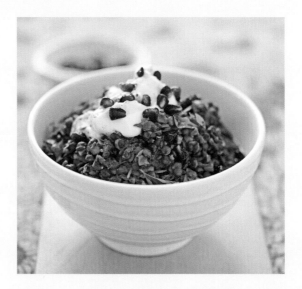

1   Preheat the slow cooker if necessary. Heat the oil in a large
    frying pan over a medium heat, add the onion and cook
    for 4–5 minutes until just beginning to soften. Stir in the
    ginger, garlic, cumin and coriander seeds.

2   Place the lentils in a sieve and rinse under cold running
    water. Drain and transfer to the slow cooker pot. Spoon the
    onion mixture on top, then add the celery and tomatoes.
    Pour over the hot stock, season to taste, cover and cook on
    High for 4–5 hours until the lentils are tender.

3   Stir in the lemon juice and herbs and spoon into bowls.
    Top with the yogurt and harissa, then scatter with the
    pomegranate seeds and serve immediately.

sweet potato & egg curry

1 tablespoon sunflower oil

1 onion, chopped

1 teaspoon cumin seeds,
   roughly crushed

1 teaspoon ground coriander

1 teaspoon ground turmeric

1 teaspoon garam masala

½ teaspoon dried chilli flakes

300 g (10 oz) sweet potatoes,
   diced

2 garlic cloves, finely chopped

400 g (13 oz) can chopped
   tomatoes

400 g (13 oz) can lentils,
   drained

300 ml (½ pint) vegetable stock

1 teaspoon caster sugar

6 hard-boiled eggs, halved

150 g (5 oz) frozen peas

150 ml (¼ pint) single cream

small bunch of fresh coriander,
   torn

salt and pepper

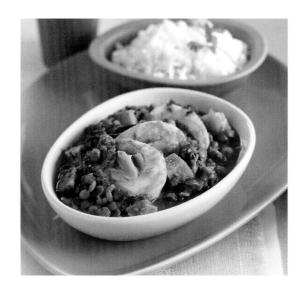

1   Preheat the slow cooker if necessary. Heat the oil in a frying
    pan over a medium heat, add the onion and cook for
    5 minutes until softened. Stir in the spices, sweet potatoes
    and garlic and cook for 2 minutes, stirring.

2   Add the tomatoes, lentils, stock and sugar and season to
    taste. Bring to the boil, stirring, then transfer to the slow
    cooker pot, cover and cook on Low for 6–8 hours until the
    sweet potatoes are tender.

3   Add the eggs to the slow cooker pot with the peas, cream and
    half the coriander. Cover again and cook for 15 minutes more.
    Serve in bowls, garnished with the remaining coriander.

for mixed vegetable curry

CALORIES PER SERVING 335

Follow the recipe above, using
100 g (3½ oz) halved fine beans
and 50 g (2 oz) shredded kale
instead of the eggs, adding them
to the slow cooker pot at the
same time as the peas.

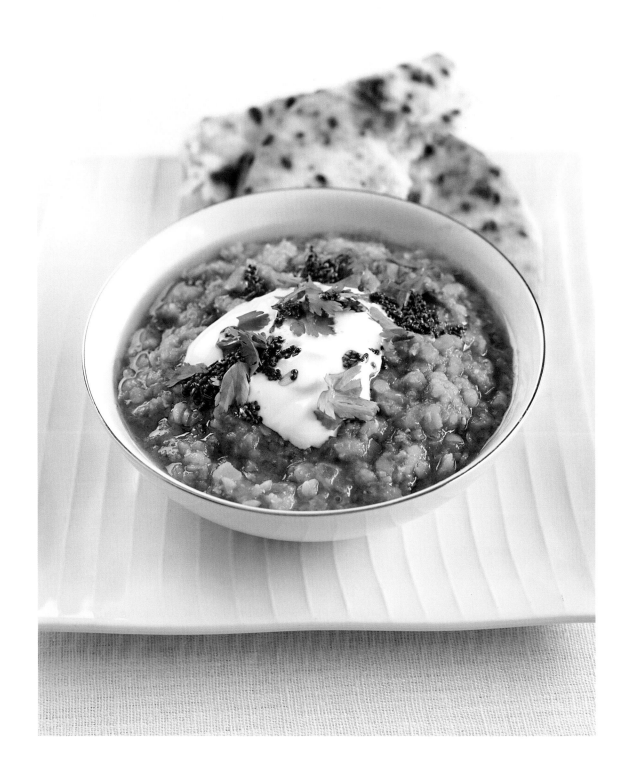

tarka dal

250 g (8 oz) dried red lentils

1 onion, finely chopped

½ teaspoon ground turmeric

½ teaspoon cumin seeds,
roughly crushed

2 cm (¾ inch) piece of fresh
root ginger, finely chopped

200 g (7 oz) can chopped
tomatoes

600 ml (1 pint) hot vegetable
stock

salt and pepper

fresh coriander leaves, torn,
to garnish

TARKA

1 tablespoon sunflower oil

2 teaspoons black mustard
seeds

½ teaspoon cumin seeds,
roughly crushed

pinch of ground turmeric

2 garlic cloves, finely chopped

TO SERVE

150 ml (¼ pint) natural yogurt

2 warm naan breads, halved

1 Preheat the slow cooker if necessary. Place the lentils in a sieve, rinse under cold running water, drain, then place in the slow cooker pot with the onion, spices, ginger, tomatoes and hot stock. Season lightly, cover and cook on High for 3-4 hours or until the lentils are soft and tender.

2 Meanwhile, heat the oil for the tarka in a small frying pan, add the remaining tarka ingredients and cook, stirring, for 2 minutes.

3 Roughly mash the lentil mixture, then spoon into bowls. Top with spoonfuls of yogurt and drizzle with the tarka. Sprinkle with the coriander leaves and serve with warm naan bread, if liked. (Calories per serving without naan 285.)

for tarka dal with spinach

CALORIES PER SERVING 295 (NOT INCLUDING NAAN)

Follow the recipe above to cook the lentils, adding 125 g (4oz) washed and roughly shredded spinach leaves for the last 15 minutes of cooking. Fry the tarka spices as above, adding ¼ teaspoon crushed dried red chilli seeds, if liked.

tomato & squash curry

25 g (1 oz) butter

1 onion, chopped

400 g (13 oz) peeled butternut
squash, diced

2 garlic cloves, finely chopped

3.5 cm (1½ inch) piece of fresh
root ginger, finely chopped

½–1 mild red chilli, deseeded
and finely chopped

4 tablespoons ready-made
korma curry paste

150 ml (¼ pint) vegetable stock

625 g (1¼ lb) plum tomatoes,
halved

50 g (2 oz) creamed coconut,
crumbled

salt and pepper

roughly chopped fresh
coriander, to garnish

1 Preheat the slow cooker if necessary. Heat the butter in a
large frying pan over a medium heat, add the onion and cook
for 5 minutes until softened. Stir in the butternut squash,
garlic, ginger and chilli, to taste, and cook for 2–3 minutes. Mix
in the curry paste and cook for 1 minute, then stir in the stock
and bring to the boil.

2 Transfer the mixture to the slow cooker pot, then arrange the
tomatoes, cut sides up, in a single layer on top. Sprinkle with
the coconut and season to taste. Cover and cook on Low for
5–6 hours or until the squash is tender and the tomatoes are
soft but still holding their shape.

3 Spoon into bowls, sprinkle with roughly chopped coriander
and serve with pilau rice, if liked.

for quick pilau rice, to serve as an accompaniment

CALORIES PER SERVING 189

Rinse 175 g (6 oz) basmati rice under cold running water, then
drain. Heat 10 g (3¾ oz) butter and 1 tablespoon sunflower oil in
a large frying pan, add 1 chopped onion and cook until softened.
Stir in 1 dried red chilli, 1 cinnamon stick, halved, 1 teaspoon cumin
seeds, 1 bay leaf, 6 crushed cardamom pods, ½ teaspoon ground
turmeric and a little salt. Add 475 ml (16 fl oz) boiling water, cover
and simmer gently for 10 minutes. Take off the heat and leave to
stand for 5–8 minutes without lifting the lid. Fluff up with a fork
before serving.

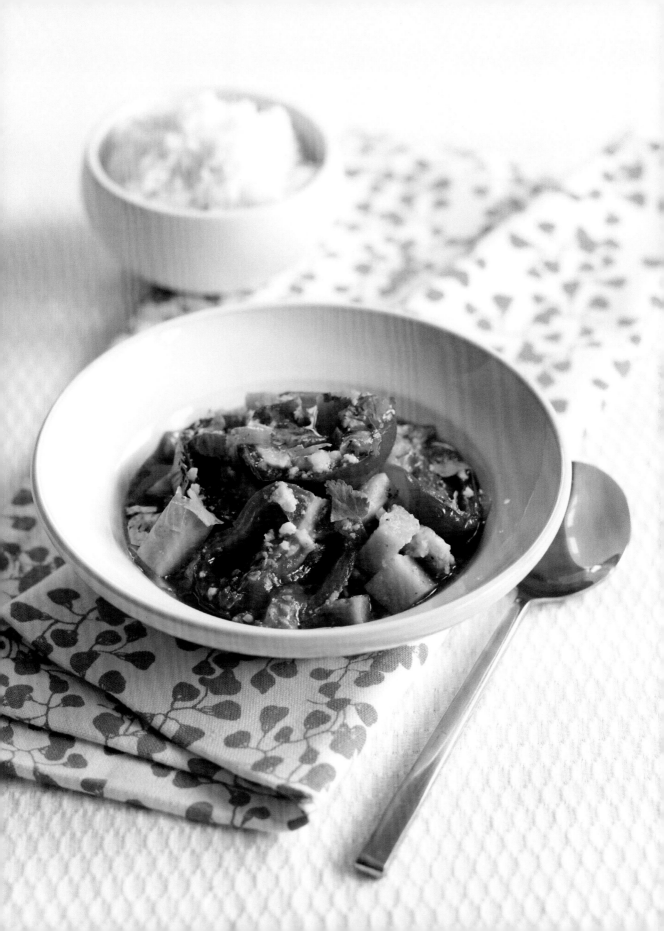

vegetable rice medley

200 g (7 oz) white basmati rice,
  soaked in cold water for 10 minutes
4 spring onions, chopped
1 red pepper, cored, deseeded
  and diced
150 g (5 oz) peeled pumpkin or
  butternut squash, cut into 1 cm
  (½ inch) dice
2 tomatoes, diced
400 g (13 oz) can black-eye beans,
  drained
leaves from 2 thyme sprigs
½-1 red chilli, deseeded
½ teaspoon ground
  allspice
½ teaspoon salt
750 ml (1¼ pints) boiling water
15 g (½ oz) fresh coriander, finely
  chopped
pepper

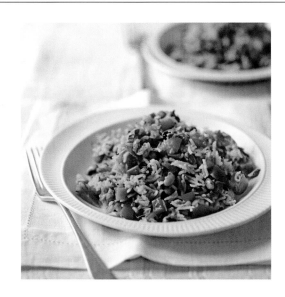

for pumpkin rice

CALORIES PER SERVING 248

Place the soaked and rinsed rice
in the slow cooker pot with the
spring onions, 375 g (12 oz) peeled
and diced pumpkin, 2 chopped
garlic cloves, leaves from 2 thyme
sprigs, 2.5 cm (1 inch) piece of fresh
root ginger, grated, and ½-1 red
chilli. Pour over 750 ml (1¼ pints)
hot water, season generously and
cook as above. Stir in the chopped
coriander just before serving.

1 Preheat the slow cooker if necessary. Place the soaked
   rice in a sieve and rinse under cold running water. Drain
   and place in the slow cooker pot with the spring onions,
   red pepper, pumpkin or butternut squash, tomatoes,
   beans, thyme and chilli, to taste.

2 Stir the allspice and salt into the boiling water and pour
   over the rice. Season generously with black pepper.
   Cover and cook on High for 1½-2 hours until the rice
   is tender and has absorbed the water, stirring once
   during cooking and adding a little more hot water if the
   rice is too dry. Add the coriander and fluff up the rice
   with a fork before serving.

mushroom & tomato rigatoni

250 g (8 oz) rigatoni or pasta
quills

3 tablespoons olive oil

1 onion, sliced

2–3 garlic cloves, finely chopped

250 g (8 oz) closed-cap
mushrooms, sliced

250 g (8 oz) portobello
mushrooms, sliced

250 g (8 oz) tomatoes, cut
into chunks

400 g (13 oz) can chopped
tomatoes

200 ml (7 fl oz) vegetable stock

1 tablespoon tomato purée

3 rosemary sprigs

salt and pepper

vegetarian Parmesan-style
cheese (optional)

for cheesy mushroom macaroni

CALORIES PER SERVING 416

Follow the recipe above, using
250 g (8 oz) macaroni instead of
the rigatoni. Mix 3 eggs with
250 ml (8 fl oz) natural yogurt,
75 g (3 oz) grated feta cheese and
a pinch of grated nutmeg. Spoon
the mixture over the top of the
mushroom and pasta mixture for
the last hour of cooking until set.
Place under a preheated hot grill
to brown the top before serving.

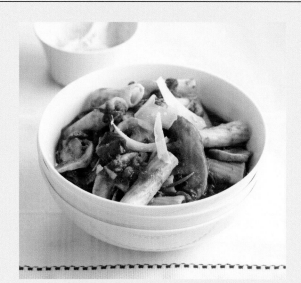

1 Preheat the slow cooker if necessary. Place the pasta in a large
bowl, cover with boiling water and leave to stand for 10 minutes.

2 Heat 1 tablespoon of the oil in a large frying pan over a medium
heat, add the onion and cook for 5 minutes, until softened.
Stir in the remaining oil, the garlic and mushrooms and cook,
stirring, until the mushrooms are just beginning to brown.

3 Stir in the fresh and canned tomatoes, stock and tomato purée.
Add the rosemary, season to taste and bring to the boil.

4 Drain the pasta and put it in the slow cooker pot. Pour over the
hot mushroom mixture and spread into an even layer. Cover
and cook on Low for 2½–3 hours or until the pasta is just tender.
Spoon into shallow bowls. Serve sprinkled with Parmesan
cheese, if liked.

HEALTHIER MAINS

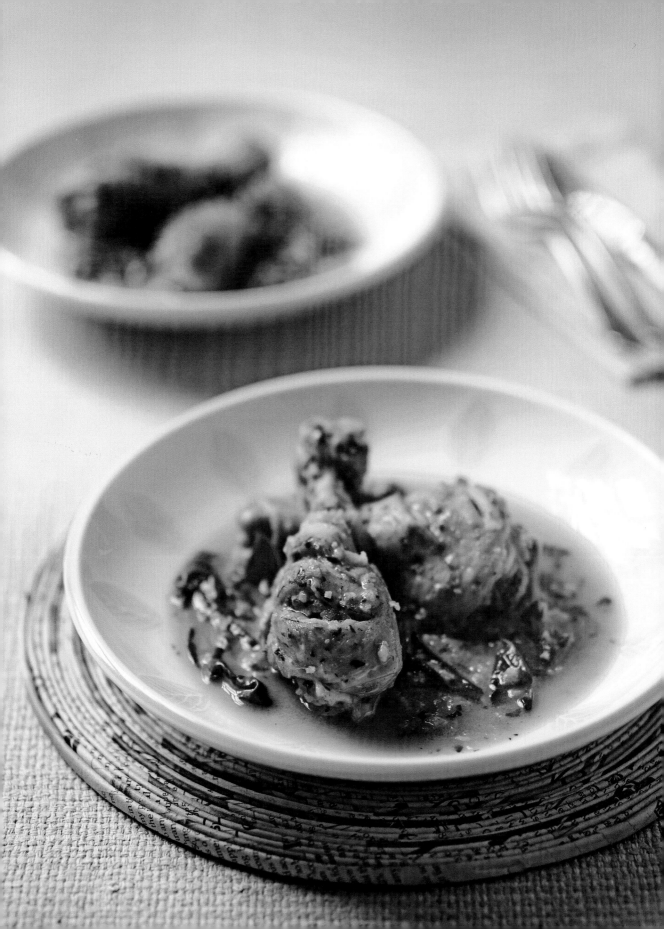

black pepper chicken

1 large onion, quartered

3 garlic cloves, halved

4 cm (1½ inch) piece of fresh
   root ginger, sliced

15 g (½ oz) fresh coriander

8 small skinless chicken
   drumsticks, 875 g (1¾ lb)
   in total

low-calorie cooking oil spray

5 cm (2 inch) cinnamon stick

1 teaspoon ground cumin

1 teaspoon ground turmeric

2 teaspoons black peppercorns,
   roughly crushed

juice of ½ lemon

350 ml (12 fl oz) chicken stock

150 g (5 oz) baby spinach

salt

1 Preheat the slow cooker if necessary. Place the onion, garlic, ginger and coriander in a food processor and blitz until very finely chopped.

2 Slash each chicken drumstick 2 or 3 times with a sharp knife. Spray a large frying pan with a little low-calorie cooking oil spray and place over a high heat until hot. Add the chicken and cook for 4–5 minutes, turning until browned all over. Transfer to the slow cooker pot, packing them in tightly together.

3 Add the chopped onion mixture to the frying pan and cook for 2 minutes until just softened. Stir in the cinnamon, cumin, turmeric and peppercorns, then add the lemon juice and stock. Season to taste and bring to the boil, stirring.

4 Pour the hot stock over the chicken, cover and cook on Low for 7–8 hours until the chicken is cooked through and beginning to shrink on the bones. Stir the sauce, add the spinach, cover again and cook on High for 15–30 minutes until the spinach has wilted. Spoon into shallow bowls and serve immediately with rice.

---

for chicken & chickpea curry

CALORIES PER SERVING 123

Follow the recipe above, using just 4 chicken drumsticks and adding ¼ teaspoon chilli powder instead of the black pepper. Place the browned drumsticks in the slow cooker pot with a 400 g (13 oz) can of chickpeas, drained, then pour over the hot stock and cook as above.

brown stew trout

4 small trout, gutted, heads
   and fins removed and well
   rinsed with cold water
1 teaspoon ground allspice
1 teaspoon paprika
1 teaspoon ground coriander
2 tablespoons olive oil
6 spring onions, thickly sliced
1 red pepper, cored, deseeded
   and thinly sliced
2 tomatoes, roughly chopped
½ red hot bonnet or other red
   chilli, deseeded and chopped
2 sprigs of thyme
300 ml (½ pint) fish stock
salt and pepper

1 Preheat the slow cooker if necessary. Slash the trout on each side 2—3 times with a sharp knife. Mix the spices and a little salt and pepper on a plate, then dip each side of the trout in the spice mix.

2 Heat the oil in a frying pan, add the trout and fry until browned on both sides but not cooked all the way through. Drain and arrange in the slow cooker pot so that they fit snugly in a single layer.

3 Add the remaining ingredients to the frying pan with any spices left on the plate and bring to the boil, stirring. Pour over the trout, then cover with the lid and cook on High for 1½—2 hours or until the fish breaks into flakes when pressed in the centre with a knife.

4 Lift the fish carefully out of the slow cooker pot using a fish slice and transfer to shallow dishes. Spoon the sauce over and serve.

for brown stew chicken

CALORIES PER SERVING 331

Use 8 chicken thigh joints instead of the trout. Slash and dip in the spice mix as above. Fry in the olive oil until browned, then drain and transfer to the slow cooker pot. Heat the vegetables as above using 450 ml (¾ pint) chicken stock instead of fish stock, season, then cook with the chicken joints in the slow cooker on Low for 8—10 hours. Thicken the sauce if liked with 4 teaspoons cornflour mixed with a little water, stir into the sauce and cook for 15 minutes more.

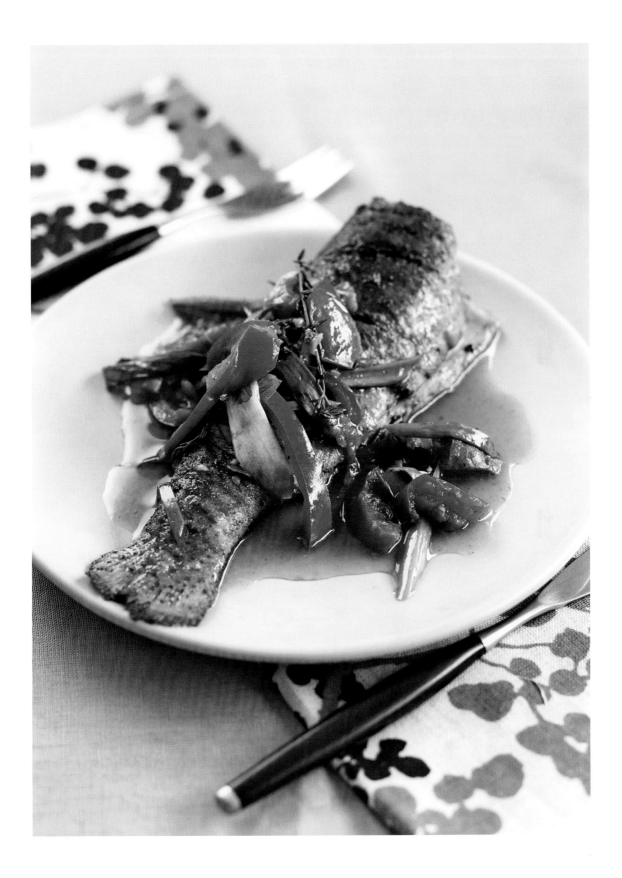

turkey kheema mutter

low-calorie cooking oil spray

500 g (1 lb) minced turkey
   breast

1 onion, chopped

2 garlic cloves, finely chopped

2.5 cm (1 inch) piece of fresh
   root ginger, finely chopped

1 teaspoon cumin seeds,
   crushed

4 teaspoons medium-hot
   curry powder

500 g (1 lb) passata

2 teaspoons granular
   sweetener

150 g (5 oz) frozen peas

4 tablespoons chopped
   fresh coriander

salt and pepper

½ red onion, thinly sliced,
   to garnish

4 small chapatis, 50 g (2 oz)
   each, to serve

1   Preheat the slow cooker if necessary. Spray a large frying
    pan with a little low-calorie cooking oil spray and place over
    a high heat until hot. Add the minced turkey and onion and
    fry for 4–5 minutes, stirring and breaking up the mince with a
    wooden spoon until it is just beginning to brown.

2   Stir in the garlic, ginger, cumin and curry powder and cook
    for 1 minute, then add the passata and sweetener. Season
    to taste and bring to the boil, stirring. Transfer to the slow
    cooker pot, cover and cook on Low for 8–10 hours until the
    turkey is cooked through.

3   Add the frozen peas to the slow cooker pot with half the
    coriander. Cover again and cook on High for 15 minutes.
    Sprinkle with the remaining coriander and the red onion
    and serve with the chapatis.

for kheema mutter jackets

CALORIES PER SERVING 399

Follow the recipe above to make and cook the turkey and pea
mixture. Scrub and prick 4 baking potatoes, 175 g (6 oz) each,
place in the microwave on a sheet of kitchen paper and cook on
full power for about 20 minutes, until tender. Transfer to serving
plates, cut in half and top with the kheema mutter, remaining
coriander and sliced red onion.

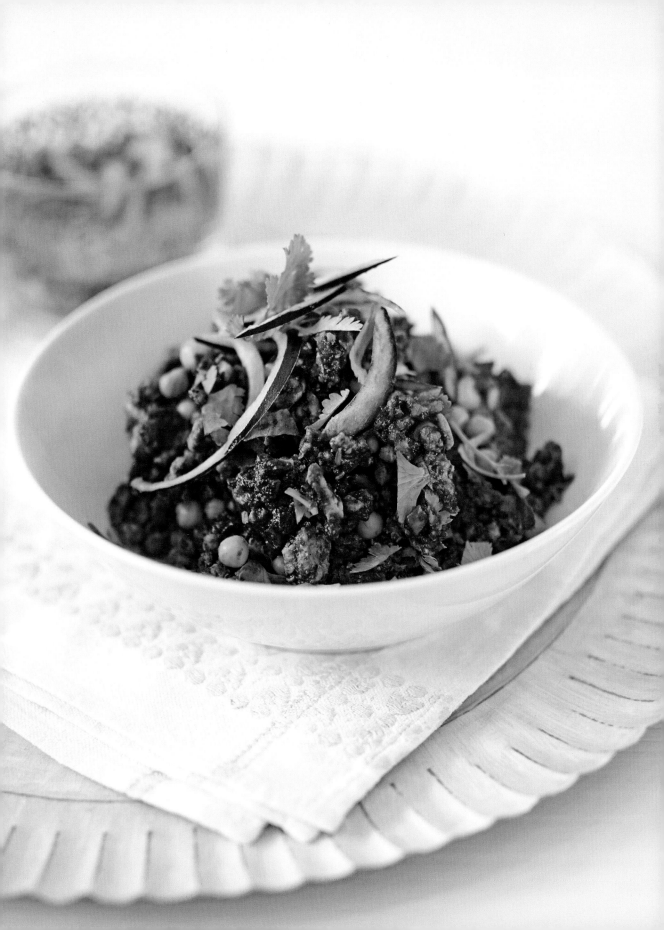

smoked cod with bean mash

2 x 400 g (13 oz) cans cannellini
   beans, drained
bunch of spring onions, thinly
   sliced
400 ml (14 fl oz) hot fish stock
1 teaspoon wholegrain mustard
grated rind and juice of 1 lemon
4 smoked cod loins, 625 g
   (1¼ lb) in total
4 tablespoons crème fraîche
small bunch of parsley,
   watercress or rocket leaves,
   roughly chopped
salt and pepper

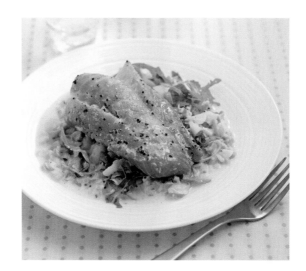

1 Preheat the slow cooker if necessary. Put the beans into the slow cooker pot with the white spring onion slices (reserving the green slices). Mix the fish stock with the mustard and lemon rind and juice, season to taste and pour into the pot.

2 Arrange the fish on top and sprinkle with a little extra pepper. Cover and cook on Low for 1½–2 hours or until the fish flakes easily when pressed with a small knife. Transfer the fish to a plate and keep warm.

3 Pour off nearly all the cooking liquid, then mash the beans roughly. Stir in the crème fraîche, the reserved green spring onion slices and the parsley, watercress or rocket. Adjust the seasoning if necessary, spoon the mash on to 4 plates and top with the fish. Serve immediately.

for baked salmon with basil bean mash

CALORIES PER SERVING 451

Follow the recipe above, omitting the mustard. Use 4 x 150 g (5 oz) salmon steaks instead of the cod and a small bunch of basil instead of the parsley, watercress or rocket leaves.

pot-roasted chicken with lemon

2 tablespoons olive oil

1.5 kg (3 lb) oven-ready chicken

1 large onion, cut into 6 wedges

500 ml (17 fl oz) dry cider

3 teaspoons Dijon mustard

2 teaspoons caster sugar

900 ml (1½ pints) hot chicken stock

3 carrots, cut into chunks

3 celery sticks, thickly sliced

1 lemon, cut into 6 wedges

6 tarragon sprigs

3 tablespoons crème fraîche

salt and pepper

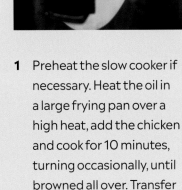

for herby pot-roasted chicken

CALORIES PER SERVING 480

Follow the recipe above, omitting the lemon and tarragon, and adding 25 g (1 oz) mixed herb sprigs, such as rosemary, sage or tarragon, and parsley or chives, to the slow cooker pot with the vegetables. Remove the herb sprigs before serving, and garnish the chicken with 3 tablespoons chopped parsley or chives.

1 Preheat the slow cooker if necessary. Heat the oil in a large frying pan over a high heat, add the chicken and cook for 10 minutes, turning occasionally, until browned all over. Transfer to the slow cooker pot, breast side down.

2 Add the onion wedges to the pan and cook over a medium heat for 3-4 minutes until lightly browned. Add the cider, mustard and sugar and season to taste. Bring to the boil, stirring, then pour over the chicken.

3 Add the hot stock, then the vegetables, lemon wedges and 3 sprigs of the tarragon, pressing the chicken and vegetables down into the liquid. Cover and cook on High for 5-6 hours or until the chicken is thoroughly cooked and the meat juices run clear when the thickest parts of the leg and breast are pierced with a sharp knife.

4 Transfer the chicken to a large serving plate and arrange the vegetables around it. Transfer 600 ml (1 pint) of the hot cooking stock to a jug. Reserve a sprig of tarragon to garnish, then chop the remainder and whisk into the jug with the crème fraîche to make a gravy. Adjust the seasoning to taste. Serve the chicken and vegetables garnished with the remaining tarragon.

minestrone soup

1 tablespoon olive oil

1 onion, chopped

1 carrot, diced

2 smoked streaky bacon rashers, chopped

2 garlic cloves, finely chopped

4 tomatoes, skinned and chopped

2 celery sticks, diced

2 small courgettes, diced

3 teaspoons ready-made pesto, plus 1 extra teaspoon to serve

1.2 litres (2 pints) chicken or vegetable stock

75 g (3 oz) purple sprouting broccoli, cut into small pieces

40 g (1½ oz) tiny soup pasta

salt and pepper

4 tablespoons freshly grated Parmesan cheese, to serve

1 Preheat the slow cooker if necessary. Heat the oil in a large frying pan over a high heat, add the onion, carrot and bacon and cook for 5 minutes, until lightly browned. Add the garlic, then stir in the tomatoes, celery and courgettes and cook for 1–2 minutes. Stir in the pesto and stock, season to taste and bring to the boil, stirring.

2 Pour into the slow cooker pot, cover and cook on Low for 6–8 hours or until the vegetables are tender. Add the broccoli and pasta, cover again and cook on High for 15–30 minutes or until the pasta is tender.

3 Stir well, taste and adjust the seasoning, if necessary, then ladle the soup into bowls. Drizzle each bowl with ½ teaspoon of pesto, to taste. Sprinkle with the grated Parmesan and serve.

---

for curried vegetable & chicken soup

CALORIES PER SERVING 255

Follow the recipe above, using 2 diced boneless, skinless chicken thighs instead of the bacon and 3 teaspoons mild curry paste instead of the pesto. Add 40 g (1½ oz) basmati rice with 1.2 litres (2 pints) chicken stock and continue as above, omitting the pasta. Garnish with chopped fresh coriander and serve with warm naan bread, if liked.

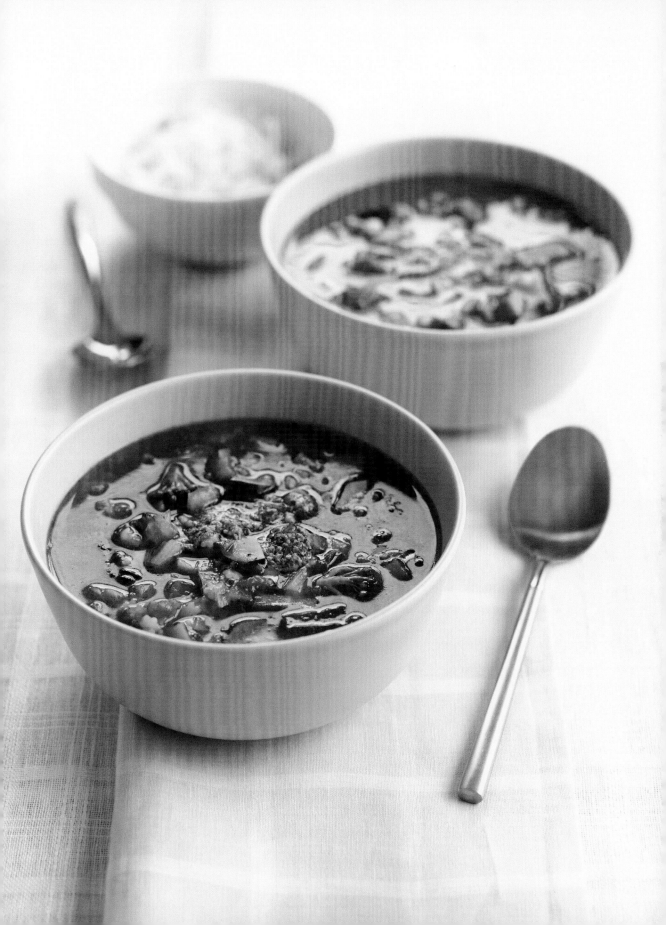

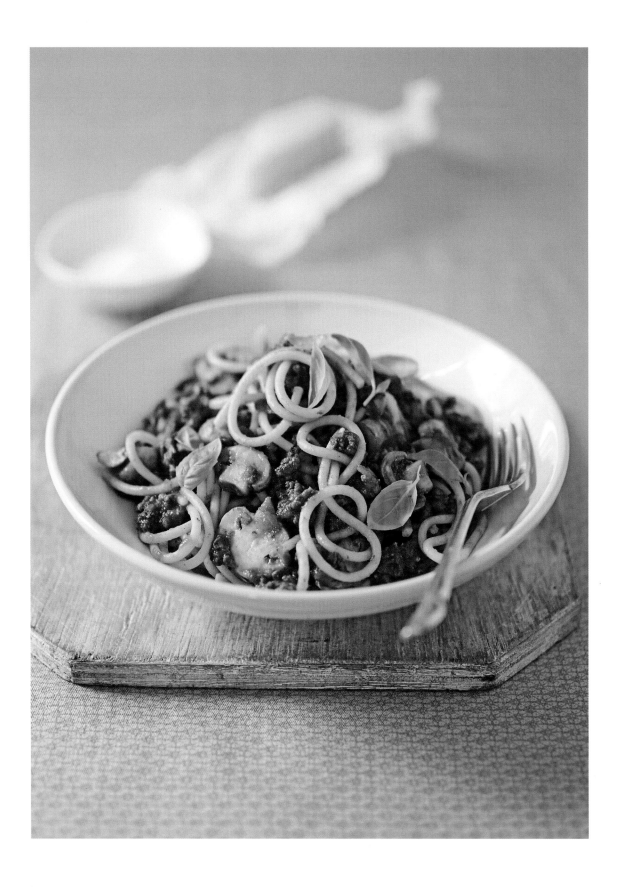

slimming spaghetti bolognese

low-calorie cooking oil spray

500 g (1 lb) extra-lean
  minced beef

1 onion, finely chopped

2 garlic cloves, finely chopped

1 carrot, coarsely grated

2 courgettes, coarsely grated

150 g (5 oz) button
  mushrooms, sliced

500 g (1 lb) passata

150 ml (¼ pint) beef stock

1 teaspoon dried oregano

salt and pepper

TO SERVE

300 g (10 oz) dried spaghetti

handful of oregano or
  basil leaves

1 Spray a large frying pan with a little low-calorie cooking oil spray and place over a high heat until hot. Add the minced beef and onion and cook for 5 minutes, stirring and breaking up the mince with a wooden spoon until evenly browned.

2 Stir in the garlic, carrot, courgette and mushrooms. Add the passata, stock and oregano, then season to taste. Bring to the boil, stirring. Transfer to the slow cooker pot, cover and cook on Low for 8–10 hours.

3 Cook the spaghetti in a large saucepan of lightly salted boiling water according to packet instructions, until tender. Drain well, toss with the Bolognese sauce and serve immediately sprinkled with oregano or basil leaves.

for tomato shepherd's pie
CALORIES PER SERVING 258

Make the Bolognese sauce as above. Peel 500 g (1 lb) potatoes and 500 g (1 lb) swede and cut into chunks. Cook in a saucepan of lightly salted boiling water for 15–20 minutes until tender. Drain and mash with 4 tablespoons vegetable stock (or 4 tablespoons cooking water). Beat 1 egg and stir half into the mash, then season to taste. Spoon the mash over the Bolognese sauce and rough up the top with a fork. Brush with the remaining beaten egg and brown under the grill before serving.

spicy salmon curry

1 onion, quartered

15 g (½ oz) fresh coriander leaves and stalks, plus extra to garnish

2.5 cm (1 inch) piece of fresh root ginger, sliced

1 lemon grass stalk, thickly sliced, or 1 teaspoon lemon grass paste

200 ml (7 fl oz) light coconut milk

200 ml (7 fl oz) fish stock

1 teaspoon Thai fish sauce

1 tablespoon Thai red curry paste

4 salmon steaks, 500 g (1 lb) in total

low-calorie cooking oil spray

400 g (13 oz) ready-prepared stir-fry vegetables

grated rind and juice of 1 lime

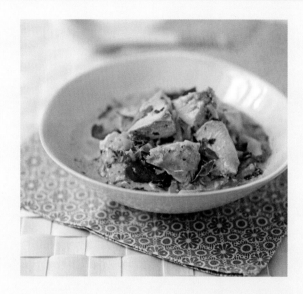

for spicy vegetable curry

CALORIES PER SERVING 138

Follow the recipe above to make the sauce, using 200 ml (7 fl oz) vegetable stock instead of the fish stock, and omitting the fish sauce if serving the curry to vegetarians. Place a 200 g (7 oz) can of bamboo shoots in the slow cooker pot with 175 g (6 oz) baby corn cobs, 150 g (5 oz) whole cherry tomatoes and 1 diced courgette. Pour over the sauce, cook and serve with stir-fried vegetables as above.

1 Preheat the slow cooker if necessary. Place the onion, coriander, ginger and lemon grass in a food processor and blitz until finely chopped. Transfer to a medium saucepan and stir in the coconut milk, stock, fish sauce and curry paste. This mixture can be chilled until ready to use.

2 Arrange the salmon steaks in the base of the slow cooker pot. Bring the coconut mixture to the boil, stirring, then pour over the salmon. Cover and cook on Low for 2–3 hours until the salmon flakes easily when pressed with a small knife.

3 Spray a large frying pan with a little low-calorie cooking oil spray and place over a high heat until hot. Add the vegetables and cook for 2–3 minutes until piping hot.

4 Break the salmon into large flakes and stir the lime rind and juice into the curry. Spoon into bowls and top with the vegetables and a little extra coriander.

hearty winter sausage stew

low-calorie cooking oil spray

50 g (2 oz) smoked back bacon, trimmed of fat and chopped

1 red onion, chopped

½ teaspoon smoked hot paprika or chilli powder

300 ml (½ pint) chicken stock

400 g (13 oz) can reduced sugar baked beans

450 g (14½ oz) extra-lean sausages

1 red pepper, cored, deseeded and chopped

400 g (13 oz) peeled pumpkin, diced

2 celery sticks, thickly sliced

2 sage sprigs or ½ teaspoon dried sage

salt and pepper

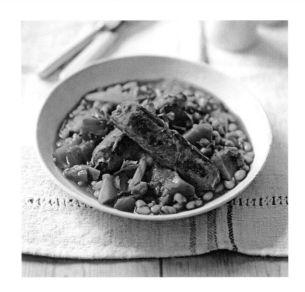

for bonfire night chicken stew

CALORIES PER SERVING 315

Follow the recipe above, using 625 g (1¼ lb) boneless, skinless chicken thighs instead of the sausages, and browning it with the bacon and onion. Add to the slow cooker pot with the vegetables, pour over the hot stock and beans, cover and cook on Low for 7–8 hours.

1   Preheat the slow cooker if necessary. Spray a large frying pan with a little low-calorie cooking oil spray and place over a high heat until hot. Add the bacon and onion and fry for 4–5 minutes, stirring until just beginning to brown. Stir in the paprika, then pour in the stock and baked beans. Season to taste, then bring to the boil, stirring.

2   Arrange the sausages in a single layer in the base of the slow cooker pot, top with the red pepper, pumpkin, celery and sage, then pour over the hot stock and beans. Cover and cook on High for 5–6 hours. Stir the stew, spoon into shallow bowls and serve.

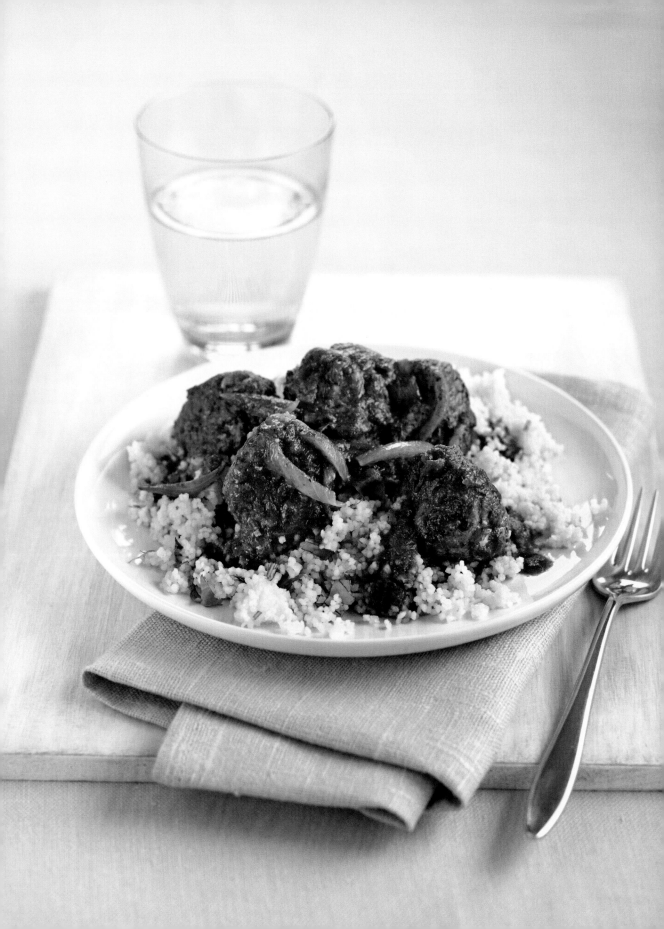

turkey meatballs

500 g (1 lb) minced turkey
  breast
100 g (3½ oz) drained canned
  green lentils
1 egg yolk
1 tablespoon olive oil
1 onion, sliced
2 garlic cloves, finely chopped
1 teaspoon ground turmeric
1 teaspoon ground coriander
½ teaspoon ground cumin
½ teaspoon ground cinnamon
2.5 cm (1 inch) piece of fresh
  root ginger, finely chopped
400 g (13 oz) can chopped
  tomatoes
150 ml (¼ pint) chicken stock
salt and pepper

1 Preheat the slow cooker if necessary. Place the turkey in a bowl with the lentils and egg yolk, season to taste and mix well. Shape the mixture into 20 small balls using wetted hands.

2 Heat the oil in a large frying pan over a high heat, add the meatballs and cook, stirring, until browned but not cooked through. Transfer to the slow cooker pot using a slotted spoon. Add the onion to the pan and cook over a medium heat for 5 minutes until softened, then stir in the garlic, spices and ginger and cook for 1 minute.

3 Stir in the tomatoes and stock, season to taste and bring to the boil, stirring. Pour over the meatballs, cover and cook on Low for 6–8 hours or until the meatballs are cooked through. Stir, then spoon into shallow bowls and serve with lemon couscous, if liked.

---

for lemon couscous
CALORIES PER SERVING 240

To serve as an accompaniment, place 200 g (7 oz) couscous in a large bowl with 450 ml (¾ pint) boiling water, the grated rind and juice of 1 lemon and 2 tablespoons olive oil. Season to taste, cover and leave to stand for 5 minutes. Fluff up with a fork and stir in a small bunch of chopped coriander.

sticky pork glaze ribs

1.25 kg (2½ lb) lean pork ribs
1 onion, cut into wedges
1 large carrot, sliced
3 bay leaves
2 tablespoons malt vinegar
low-calorie cooking oil spray
salt and pepper

GLAZE
8 tablespoons passata
3 tablespoons soy sauce
½ teaspoon ground cinnamon
½ teaspoon ground allspice
¼ teaspoon chilli powder
1 tablespoon dark muscovado
　sugar
grated rind and juice of
　½ orange
4 spring onions, finely chopped

1 Preheat the slow cooker if necessary. Place the pork ribs, onion and carrot in the slow cooker pot and add the bay leaves and vinegar. Season generously, then pour over enough boiling water to cover the ribs, making sure the level is at least 2.5 cm (1 inch) from the top of the pot. Cover and cook on High for 5–6 hours until the meat is starting to fall away from the bones. Transfer the ribs to a foil-lined grill pan or baking sheet.

2 Mix together the glaze ingredients, then brush all over the ribs. Spray with a little low-calorie cooking oil spray and cook under a preheated hot grill, with the ribs about 5 cm (2 inches) away from the heat, for about 10 minutes, turning from time to time and brushing with the pan juices until a deep brown. Serve with salad, if liked.

for sticky hoisin ribs
CALORIES PER SERVING 436

Follow the recipe above to cook the ribs in the slow cooker. Make a glaze by mixing together 3 tablespoons hoisin sauce, 8 tablespoons passata, ¼ teaspoon chilli powder, grated rind and juice of ½ orange and 4 finely chopped spring onions. Brush over the ribs and grill as above.

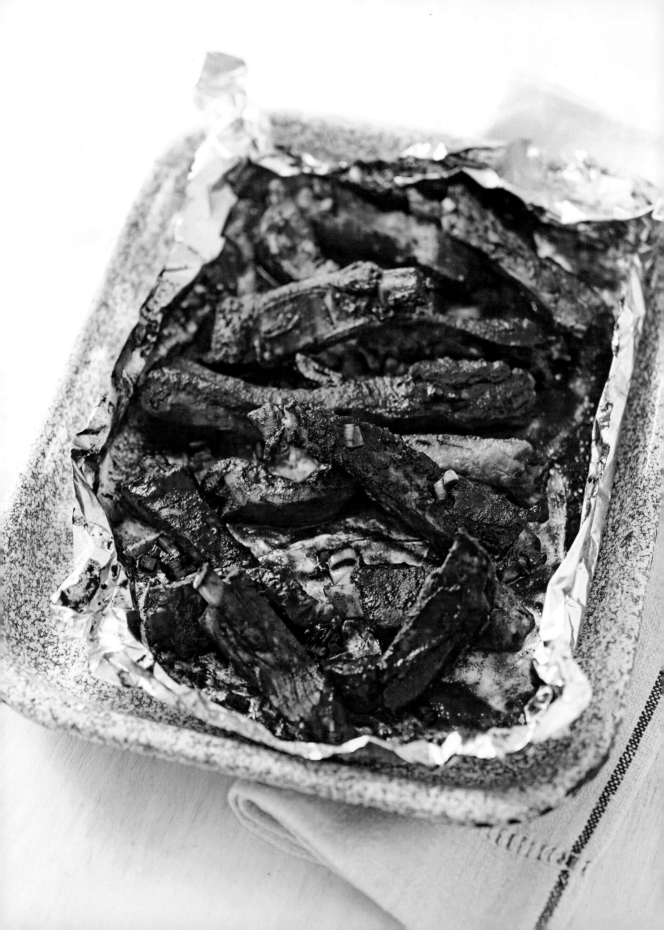

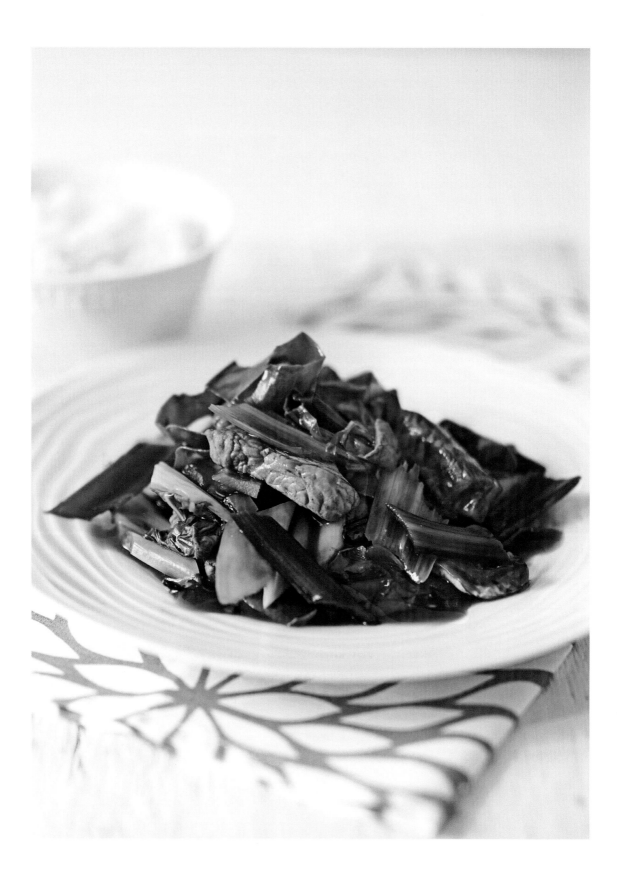

turkey with rainbow chard

low-calorie cooking oil spray

500 g (1 lb) turkey breast,
  diced

1 onion, chopped

2 garlic cloves, finely chopped

200 g (7 oz) closed-cap
  mushrooms, sliced

450 ml (¾ pint) chicken stock

2.5 cm (1 inch) piece of fresh
  root ginger, chopped

2 tablespoons soy sauce

1 tablespoon tamarind paste

1 tablespoon tomato purée

1 tablespoon cornflour

200 g (7 oz) rainbow chard,
  thickly sliced

1   Preheat the slow cooker if necessary. Spray a large frying pan with a little low-calorie cooking oil spray and place over a high heat until hot. Add the turkey, a few pieces at a time until all the turkey is in the pan, and cook for 5 minutes, stirring, until golden. Transfer to the slow cooker pot using a slotted spoon.

2   Add a little extra low-calorie cooking oil spray to the frying pan, if necessary, and cook the onion for 4–5 minutes until softened. Stir in the garlic and mushrooms and cook for 2–3 minutes more. Add the stock, ginger, soy sauce, tamarind and tomato purée, season to taste and bring to the boil, stirring. Pour over the turkey, cover and cook on Low for 8–9 hours until the turkey is cooked through.

3   Mix the cornflour to a smooth paste with a little cold water and stir into the turkey mixture. Arrange the chard on top, cover again and cook on High for 15–30 minutes until tender. Spoon into bowls and serve with rice or noodles, if liked.

for black bean turkey

CALORIES PER SERVING 294

Follow the recipe above to brown the turkey and fry the onion. Add the mushrooms to the frying pan with a 500 g (1 lb) jar of black bean cooking sauce and bring to the boil. Transfer to the slow cooker pot and cook as above. Stir-fry 275 g (9 oz) ready-prepared stir-fry vegetables in a little low-calorie cooking oil spray to serve with the turkey.

green olive-topped cod

200 g (7 oz) passata

200 g (7 oz) spinach, rinsed and drained

175 g (6 oz) tomatoes, roughly chopped

50 g (2 oz) chorizo, diced

4 skinless cod steaks, 150 g (5 oz) each

85 g (3 oz) green olives stuffed with hot pimento

small handful of basil leaves, plus extra to garnish

salt and pepper

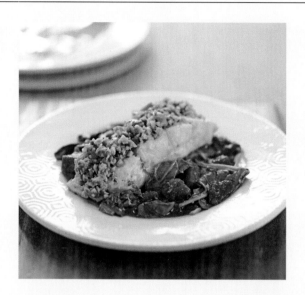

1 Preheat the slow cooker if necessary. Spoon the passata over the base of the slow cooker pot, then arrange the spinach, tomatoes and chorizo in an even layer on top. Season to taste and place the fish steaks on top in a single layer, then season again.

2 Place the olives and basil in a food processor and blitz until finely chopped, or chop with a knife. Spread the mixture over the cod steaks, then cover and cook on Low for 3½–4 hours until the fish is bright white and flakes easily when pressed with a small knife. Serve garnished with extra basil.

for herb-topped cod

CALORIES PER SERVING 249

Mix 15 g (½ oz) finely chopped parsley and 15 g (½ oz) finely chopped basil with ½ teaspoon crushed cumin seeds and the grated rind of 1 lemon. Follow the recipe above, using this herb mixture to spread over the cod steaks before cooking instead of the olives and basil.

chunky beef & barley broth

300 g (10 oz) lean stewing
   beef, diced
250 g (8 oz) swede, finely diced
250 g (8 oz) carrot, finely diced
1 onion, finely chopped
50 g (2 oz) pearl barley
50 g (2 oz) dried red lentils
900 ml (1½ pints) hot
   beef stock
1 teaspoon dried mixed herbs
1 teaspoon mustard powder
1 tablespoon Worcestershire
   sauce
125 g (4 oz) green cabbage,
   thinly shredded
salt and pepper

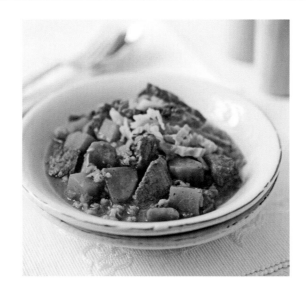

for chicken & barley broth

CALORIES PER SERVING 243

Follow the recipe above, using 300 g (10 oz) boneless, skinless diced chicken thighs and 1 sliced leek instead of the beef and onion. Use 900 ml (1½ pints) chicken stock instead of the beef stock, and 50 g (2 oz) diced stoned prunes instead of the Worcestershire sauce. Cook as above, adding the cabbage for the last 15 minutes.

1   Preheat the slow cooker if necessary. Place the beef, swede, carrot and onion in the slow cooker pot, then add the pearl barley and lentils.

2   Mix the hot stock with the herbs, mustard powder and Worcestershire sauce, then pour over the meat and vegetables. Stir well, season to taste, cover and cook on High for 5–6 hours until the beef and barley are tender.

3   Stir, then add the cabbage. Cover again and cook for 15 minutes until the cabbage is just tender. Ladle into bowls and serve.

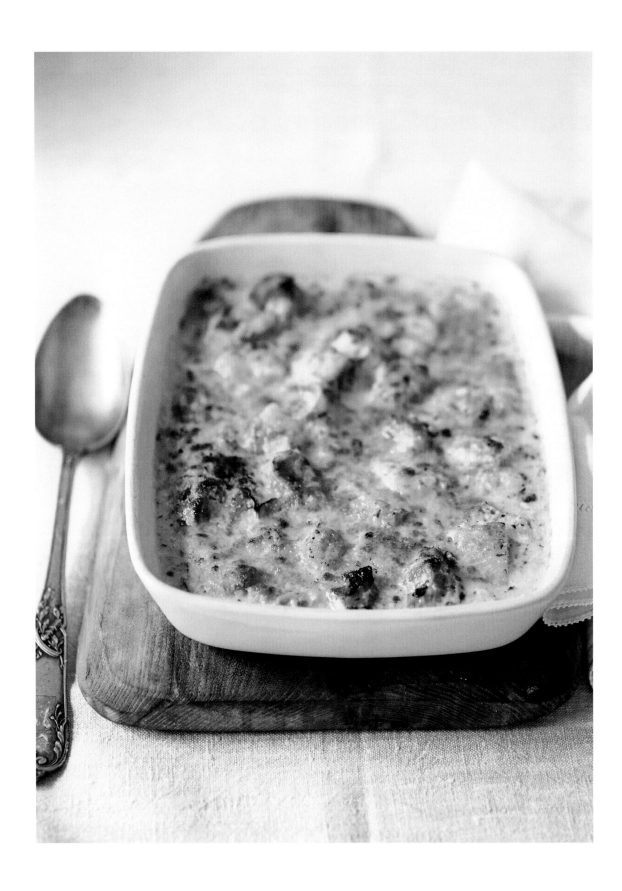

three-fish gratin

2 tablespoons cornflour

400 ml (14 fl oz) skimmed milk

50 g (2 oz) mature Cheddar
   cheese, grated

3 tablespoons chopped parsley

1 leek, thinly sliced

1 bay leaf

500 g (1 lb) mixed fish, diced
   (such as salmon, cod and
   smoked haddock)

salt and pepper

TOPPING

20 g (¾ oz) fresh breadcrumbs

40 g (1½ oz) mature Cheddar
   cheese, grated

TO SERVE

325 g (11 oz) each of peas and
   mangetout, steamed

1 Preheat the slow cooker if necessary. Place the cornflour in a saucepan with a little of the milk and mix to a smooth paste. Stir in the rest of the milk, then add the cheese, parsley, leek and bay leaf. Season to taste and bring to the boil, stirring until thickened.

2 Place the fish in the slow cooker pot. Pour over the hot leek sauce, cover and cook on Low for 2–3 hours until the fish is cooked through.

3 Transfer the fish mixture to a shallow ovenproof dish, sprinkle the breadcrumbs and cheese over the top, then place under a preheated hot grill for 4–5 minutes until golden brown. Serve with the steamed peas and mangetout.

---

for fish pies

CALORIES PER SERVING 435

Follow the recipe above, omitting the breadcrumb and cheese topping. Peel and cut 625 g (1¼ lb) potatoes into chunks. Cook the potatoes in a saucepan of lightly salted boiling water for 15 minutes or until tender. Drain and mash with 4 tablespoons skimmed milk, then season and stir in 40 g (1½ oz) grated mature Cheddar cheese. Divide the cooked fish mixture between 4 individual pie dishes, spoon over the mash, rough up the top with a fork, then brush with 1 beaten egg. Cook under a preheated medium grill until golden.

black bean & ham stew

1 onion, chopped
2 celery sticks, thickly sliced
150 g (5 oz) carrots, diced
375 g (12 oz) can black beans,
   drained
1 red chilli, halved and
   deseeded
2 thyme sprigs
pared rind of 1 orange
500 g (1 lb) unsmoked
   gammon joint, trimmed of fat
1 teaspoon mild paprika
½ teaspoon ground allspice
450 ml (¾ pint) hot
   vegetable stock
salt and pepper
4 tablespoons chopped
   parsley, to garnish

TO SERVE
150 g (5 oz) rice

1   Preheat the slow cooker if necessary. Place the onion, celery and carrot in the slow cooker pot, then add the drained beans, chilli, thyme and orange rind. Nestle the gammon joint in the centre.

2   Stir the paprika and allspice into the hot stock, then season to taste and pour over the gammon joint. Spoon some of the orange rind and thyme on top of the joint, cover and cook on High for 5–6 hours until the gammon is very tender.

3   Cook the rice in a saucepan of lightly salted boiling water, according to packet instructions, until tender.

4   Cut the gammon into pieces, then spoon into shallow bowls with the beans, vegetables and sauce. Sprinkle with the parsley and serve with the rice.

---

for black bean & chicken stew
CALORIES PER SERVING 318

Follow the recipe above, using a 1.35 kg (2 lb 10 oz) oven-ready chicken instead of the gammon joint. Cook on High for 5–6 hours or until the chicken is thoroughly cooked and the meat juices run clear when the thickest parts of the leg and breast are pierced with a sharp knife.

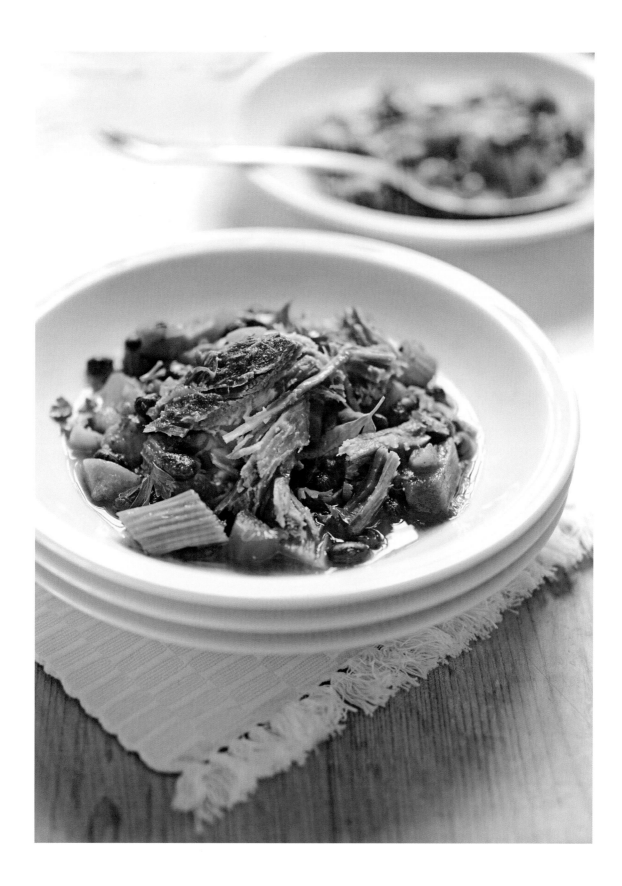

lamb & barley broth

25 g (1 oz) butter

1 tablespoon sunflower oil

1 lamb rump chop or 125 g
  (4 oz) lamb fillet, diced

1 onion, chopped

1 small leek, chopped

500 g (1 lb) mixed parsnip,
  swede, turnip and carrot, cut
  into small dice

50 g (2 oz) pearl barley

1.2 litres (2 pints) lamb or
  chicken stock

¼ teaspoon ground allspice

2-3 rosemary sprigs

salt and pepper

chopped parsley or chives,
  to garnish

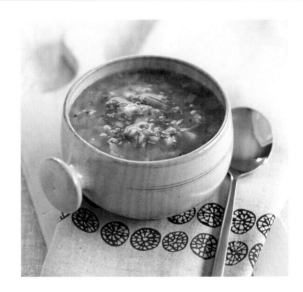

1 Preheat the slow cooker if necessary. Heat the butter and oil in a large frying pan over a high heat, add the lamb, onion and leek and cook, stirring, for 5 minutes until the lamb is lightly browned.

for lamb & dill broth
CALORIES PER SERVING 258

Follow the recipe above, adding 1 teaspoon smoked paprika, 50 g (2 oz) long-grain rice and a few sprigs of dill instead of the pearl barley. Stir in 1.2 litres (2 pints) lamb stock, 2 tablespoons red wine vinegar and 1 tablespoon light muscovado sugar. Season to taste, bring to the boil and continue as above. Garnish with chopped dill and serve with rye bread, if liked.

2 Stir in the root vegetables and barley, then add the stock, allspice and rosemary. Season to taste and bring to the boil, stirring. Pour into the slow cooker pot, cover and cook on Low for 8-10 hours or until the barley is tender.

3 Stir well, taste and adjust the seasoning, if necessary, then ladle the soup into bowls. Garnish with chopped herbs and serve.

chunky chicken & basil stew

low-calorie cooking oil spray

625 g (1¼ lb) boneless, skinless chicken thighs, each cut into 3 pieces

1 onion, chopped

2 small carrots, finely diced

2 teaspoons plain flour

350 ml (12 fl oz) chicken stock

15 g (½ oz) basil leaves, torn, plus extra to garnish

100 g (3½ oz) frozen peas, defrosted

200 g (7 oz) sprouting broccoli, stems cut into 3 or 4 pieces

150 g (5 oz) fine green beans, thickly sliced

salt and pepper

for chunky chicken with 30 garlic cloves

CALORIES PER SERVING 225

Brown 625 g (1¼ lb) boneless, skinless chicken thighs, each cut into 3 pieces, in a frying pan and place in the slow cooker pot with 30 unpeeled garlic cloves. Follow the recipe above, using 250 g (8 oz) small peeled shallots instead of the onion and carrot, and 3 thyme sprigs and 2 teaspoons Dijon mustard instead of the basil. Cook as above, omitting the green vegetables, and serve sprinkled with chopped parsley.

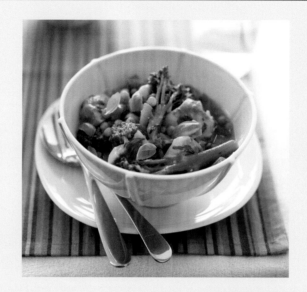

1 Preheat the slow cooker if necessary. Spray a large frying pan with a little low-calorie cooking oil spray and place over a high heat until hot. Add the chicken, a few pieces at a time until all the chicken is in the pan, and cook for 5 minutes, stirring, until golden. Transfer to the slow cooker pot using a slotted spoon.

2 Add a little more low-calorie cooking oil spray to the pan if necessary, then cook the onion for 4–5 minutes until just beginning to soften. Stir in the carrots and flour, then add the stock and bring to the boil, stirring.

3 Add the basil, season to taste and pour over the chicken. Cover and cook on Low for 8–10 hours until the chicken is tender and cooked through. Add the peas, broccoli and green beans, cover again and cook on High for 15–30 minutes until the vegetables are tender. Serve in shallow bowls, garnished with extra basil.

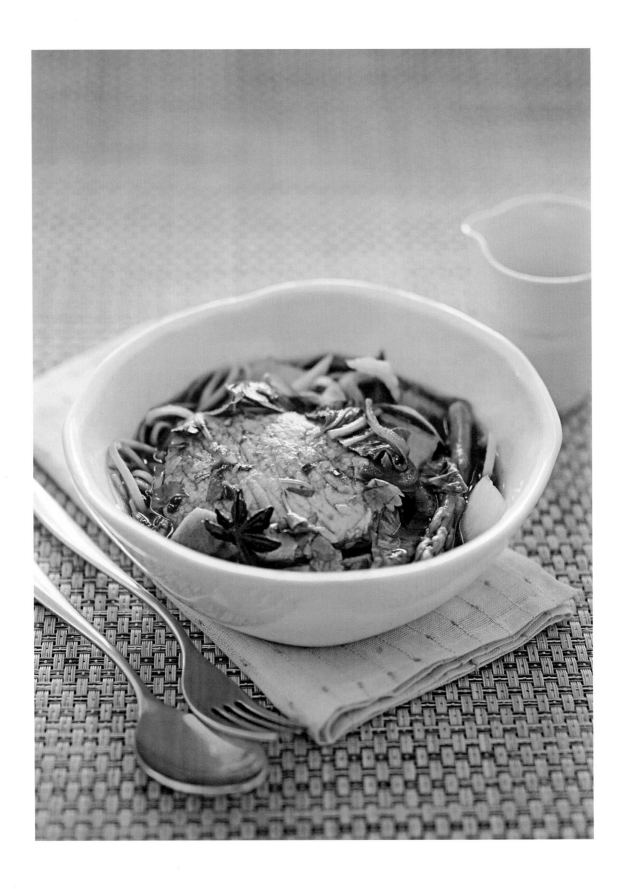

spiced pork with pak choi

4 pork medallions, 350 g
(11½ oz) in total
1 red onion, thinly sliced
2.5 cm (1 inch) piece of fresh
root ginger, thinly sliced
1 garlic clove, thinly sliced
small handful of fresh
coriander leaves
¼ teaspoon dried chilli flakes
2 small star anise
1 teaspoon Thai fish sauce
2 teaspoons tomato purée
4 teaspoons dark soy sauce
350 ml (12 fl oz) hot chicken
stock
200 g (7 oz) pak choi, thickly
sliced
100 g (3½ oz) asparagus tips
250 g (8 oz) dried egg noodles,
to serve

1 Preheat the slow cooker if necessary. Place the pork medallions in the slow cooker pot in a single layer and scatter with the onion, ginger and garlic. Sprinkle half the coriander leaves on top.

2 Stir the chilli flakes, star anise, fish sauce, tomato purée and soy sauce into the hot chicken stock, then pour over the pork. Cover and cook on Low for 6–7 hours until the pork is tender.

3 Add the pak choi and asparagus to the slow cooker pot, cover and cook on High for 15 minutes until the vegetables are just tender and still bright green.

4 Meanwhile, cook the egg noodles in a saucepan of lightly salted boiling water according to packet instructions until tender. Drain and divide between 4 bowls, top with the pork and vegetables, then spoon over the broth and serve garnished with the remaining coriander.

---

for spiced pork with mixed vegetables
CALORIES PER SERVING 409

Follow the recipe above, adding 300 g (10 oz) ready-prepared mixed stir-fry vegetables instead of the pak choi and asparagus.

chilli turkey tortillas

low-calorie cooking oil spray

400 g (13 oz) minced turkey breast

1 onion, chopped

2 garlic cloves, finely chopped

1 teaspoon dried chilli flakes

1 teaspoon cumin seeds, crushed

1 teaspoon mild paprika

400 g (13 oz) can chopped tomatoes

200 g (7 oz) can red kidney beans, drained

150 ml (¼ pint) chicken stock

1 tablespoon tomato purée

1 red pepper, cored, deseeded and diced

TO SERVE

4 x 20 cm (8 inch) soft tortilla wraps, 40 g (1½ oz) each

50 g (2 oz) salad leaves

4 tablespoons 0% fat Greek yogurt

40 g (1½ oz) reduced-fat Cheddar cheese, grated

fresh coriander, torn

1 Preheat the slow cooker if necessary. Spray a large frying pan with a little low-calorie cooking oil spray and place over a high heat until hot. Add the minced turkey and onion and fry for 4–5 minutes, stirring and breaking up the mince with a wooden spoon until it is just beginning to brown.

2 Stir in the garlic, chilli, cumin seeds and paprika, then add the tomatoes, kidney beans, stock and tomato purée. Add the red pepper, season to taste and bring to the boil. Transfer to the slow cooker pot, cover and cook on Low for 8–10 hours until the turkey is cooked through.

3 Warm the tortillas in a hot dry frying pan for 1–2 minutes each side, then place on 4 serving plates. Spoon the spicy turkey on top, then add a handful of salad leaves to each, a spoonful of yogurt, a little Cheddar and some torn coriander. Serve immediately.

---

for turkey with a mashed potato topping

CALORIES PER SERVING 440

Follow the recipe above to make and cook the turkey mixture. Cook, drain and mash 750 g (1½ lb) potatoes, stir in 4 tablespoons vegetable stock and season to taste. Place the turkey mixture in a shallow heatproof dish and spoon the mashed potato on top. Rough up the top with a fork, then brush with ½ beaten egg. Brown under the grill before serving.

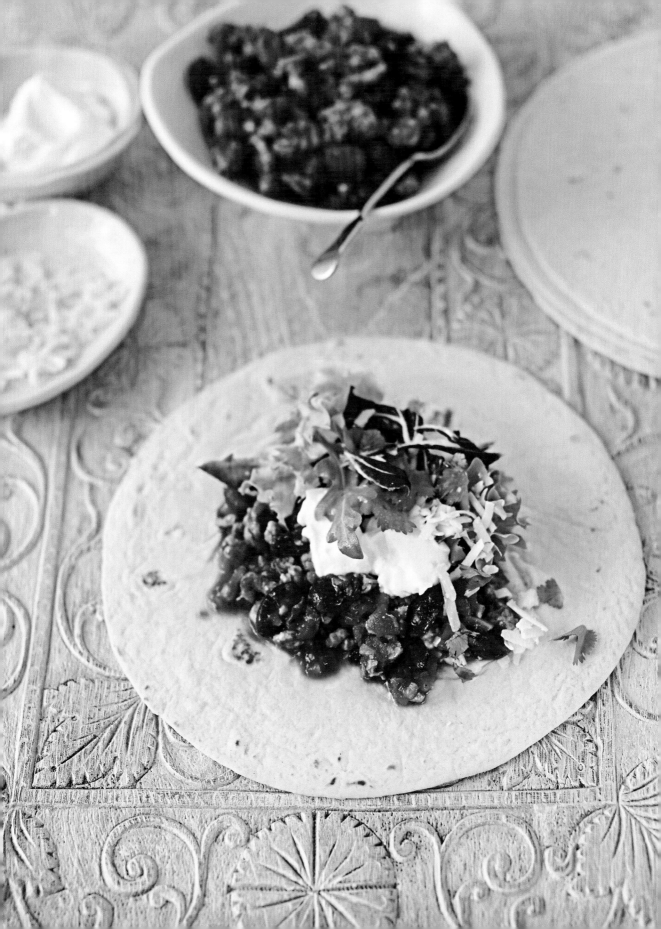

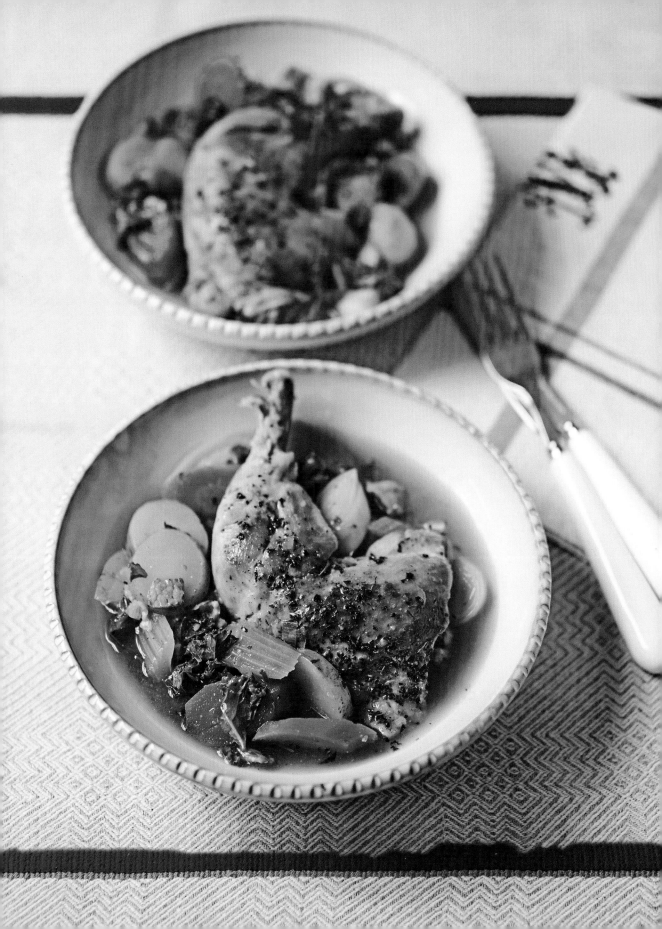

all-in-one chicken casserole

low-calorie cooking oil spray

4 skinless chicken legs, 875 g (1¾ lb) in total

50 g (2 oz) smoked back bacon, trimmed of fat and chopped

300 g (10 oz) baby new potatoes, thickly sliced

2 small leeks, thickly sliced

2 celery sticks, thickly sliced

2 carrots, sliced

2 teaspoons plain flour

1 teaspoon dried mixed herbs

1 teaspoon mustard powder

450 ml (¾ pint) chicken stock

50 g (2 oz) curly kale, sliced

salt and pepper

1   Spray a large frying pan with a little low-calorie cooking oil spray and place over a high heat until hot. Add the chicken and cook for 5 minutes, turning, until browned all over. Transfer to the slow cooker pot.

2   Add the bacon and potatoes to the frying pan with a little extra low-calorie cooking oil spray and cook for 4–5 minutes, stirring, until the bacon is beginning to brown. Stir in the white leek slices (reserving the green slices), the celery and carrots. Add the flour, herbs and mustard and stir well.

3   Pour in the stock, season to taste and bring to the boil, stirring. Spoon over the chicken, cover and cook on Low for 8–10 hours or until the chicken is thoroughly cooked and the meat juices run clear when the thickest parts of the leg are pierced with a sharp knife.

4   Add the reserved green leek slices and the kale to the slow cooker pot, cover and cook for 15 minutes until the vegetables are just tender. Serve in shallow bowls.

for chicken hotpot
CALORIES PER SERVING 403

Follow the main recipe to make the chicken mixture, omitting the new potatoes and carrots. Transfer to the slow cooker pot and cover with 300 g (10 oz) scrubbed and thinly sliced baking potatoes and 2 thinly sliced carrots, arranging the slices alternately overlapping. Spray with low-calorie cooking oil spray, season to taste, then cook as above. After cooking, brown the top under the grill, if liked.

corn & smoked cod chowder

low-calorie cooking oil spray

1 leek, thinly sliced

50 g (2 oz) smoked back bacon,
   trimmed of fat and diced

200 g (7 oz) potato,
   finely diced

175 g (6 oz) celeriac,
   finely diced

75 g (3 oz) frozen sweetcorn
   kernels

450 ml (¾ pint) fish stock

1 bay leaf

250 g (8 oz) smoked cod fillet

200 ml (7 fl oz) skimmed milk

50 g (2 oz) reduced-fat
   cream cheese

salt and pepper

chopped parsley, to garnish

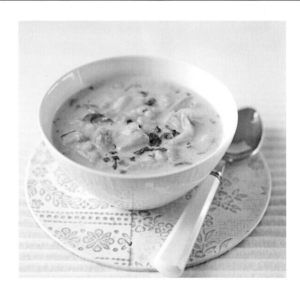

1 Preheat the slow cooker if necessary. Spray a large frying pan with a little low-calorie cooking oil spray and place over a medium heat until hot. Add the white leek slices (reserving the green slices) and the bacon and cook for 3–4 minutes until the leeks have softened and the bacon is just beginning to brown.

2 Add the potato, celeriac, sweetcorn and stock. Bring to the boil, stirring, then add the bay leaf and season to taste. Transfer to the slow cooker pot, arrange the fish on top and press the fish into the liquid. Cover and cook on High for 2–3 hours until the potatoes and celeriac are tender and the fish flakes easily when pressed with a small knife. Transfer the fish to a plate, remove the skin and bones and break into pieces.

for salmon & crab chowder

CALORIES PER SERVING 249

Follow the recipe above, using 250 g (8 oz) salmon fillet instead of the smoked cod. Cook as above, stirring in a 40 g (1½ oz) can of dark crab meat for the last 15 minutes of cooking time.

3 Stir the milk and cream cheese into the slow cooker pot, then stir in the reserved green leek slices and the flaked fish. Cover again and cook for 15 minutes until the leeks are tender. Ladle into bowls and serve garnished with the chopped parsley.

beery beef cheeks

1 tablespoon sunflower oil

600 g (1 lb 4 oz) beef cheeks, cut into 4 cm (1½ inch) thick slices

2 red onions, cut into wedges

250 ml (8 fl oz) brown ale

150 ml (¼ pint) beef stock

1 tablespoon tomato purée

2 teaspoons cornflour

2 rosemary sprigs

2 bay leaves

300 g (10 oz) small Chantenay carrots, halved lengthways

2 celery sticks, thickly sliced

salt and pepper

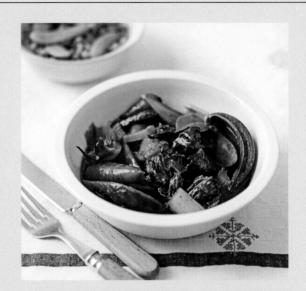

1 Heat the oil in a large frying pan over a high heat until hot. Add the beef, a few pieces at a time until all the beef is in the pan, and cook for 5 minutes, stirring until browned. Use a slotted spoon to transfer the beef to the slow cooker pot, arranging it in a single layer.

2 Add the onion to the frying pan and cook for 3–4 minutes until softened. Add the brown ale, stock and tomato purée. Mix the cornflour to a smooth paste with a little cold water and stir into the pan with the herbs. Season to taste and bring to the boil, stirring.

3 Place the carrots and celery on top of the beef, then pour over the hot beer mixture. Cover and cook on High for 5–6 hours until the beef is very tender. Spoon into shallow bowls and serve with sugar snap peas and frozen peas, if liked.

for beery chestnuts & mushrooms

CALORIES PER SERVING 219

Follow the recipe above, using 500 g (1 lb) whole mixed small mushrooms instead of the beef, and adding 175 g (6 oz) canned chestnuts at the same time as the herbs.

tandoori chicken

150 ml (¼ pint) 0% fat
   Greek yogurt

4 cm (1½ inch) piece of fresh
   root ginger, grated

3 tablespoons chopped fresh
   coriander leaves

3 teaspoons medium-hot
   curry powder

½ teaspoon ground turmeric

1 teaspoon paprika

625 g (1¼ lb) boneless,
   skinless chicken thighs, cut
   into chunks

juice of ½ lemon

low-calorie cooking oil spray

salt and pepper

TO SERVE

50 g (2 oz) mixed green salad
   leaves

¼ cucumber, diced

small handful of fresh
   coriander leaves

juice of ½ lemon

1 Place the yogurt in a mixing bowl and stir in the ginger, coriander, curry powder, turmeric and paprika. Toss the chicken with the lemon juice, season lightly and stir into the yogurt mixture until evenly coated. Cover the bowl and chill overnight.

2 Preheat the slow cooker if necessary. Stir the chicken mixture, then transfer to the slow cooker pot in an even layer. Cover and cook on High for 3–4 hours or until the chicken is tender and cooked through. (The yogurt will separate during cooking but this will not affect the taste.)

3 Spray a large frying pan with a little low-calorie cooking oil spray and place over a high heat until hot. Transfer the chicken to the frying pan, a few pieces at a time until all the chicken is in the pan, and cook for 2–3 minutes, turning once, until golden on both sides. This step can be omitted if you are short of time.

4 Toss the salad leaves, cucumber and coriander leaves with the lemon juice, arrange on serving plates and top with the chicken.

---

for garlicky tandoori chicken
CALORIES PER SERVING 209

Add 3 finely chopped garlic cloves to the yogurt and spice mixture and continue as above.

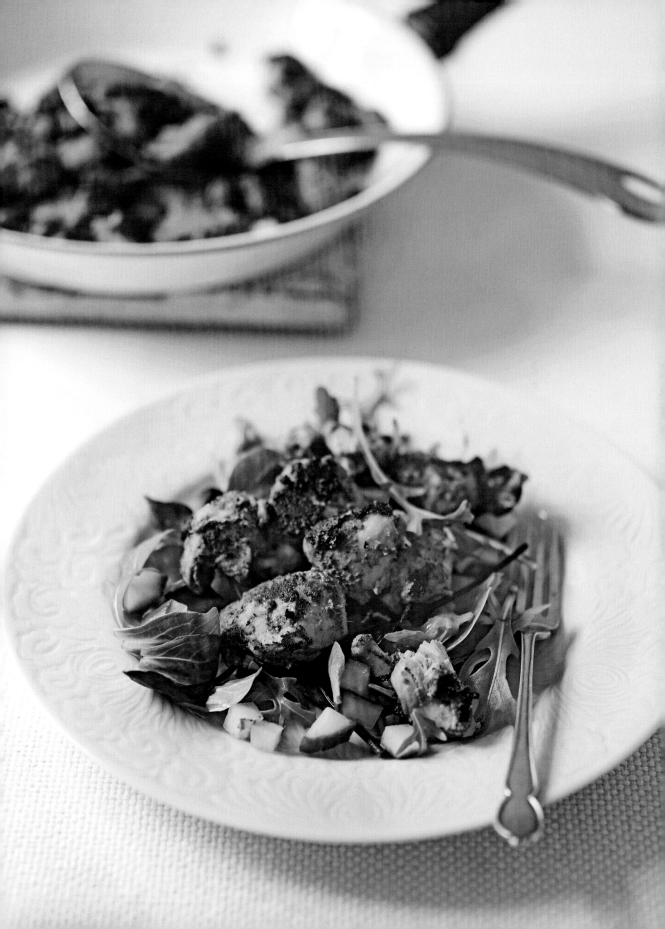

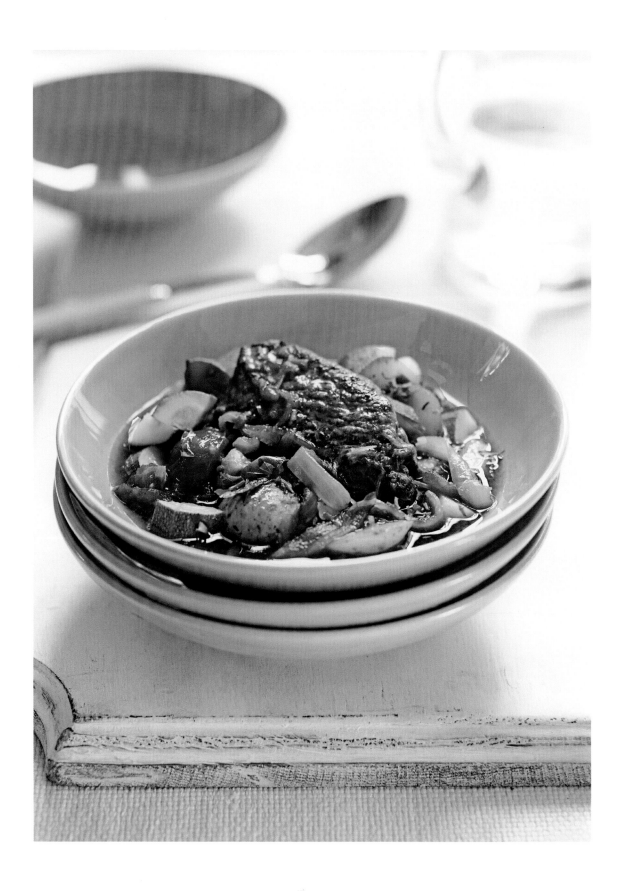

slow-cooked lamb steaks

low-calorie cooking oil spray

4 lean lamb leg steaks,

125 g (4 oz) each

1 large onion, thinly sliced

2 garlic cloves, finely chopped

1 lemon, diced

250 g (8 oz) tomatoes,
  roughly chopped

2 teaspoons coriander seeds,
  roughly crushed

1 bay leaf

1 teaspoon granular sweetener

1 tablespoon sun-dried tomato
  paste

300 ml (½ pint) lamb stock

300 g (10 oz) baby new
  potatoes, thickly sliced

300 g (10 oz) courgettes, diced

salt and pepper

2 tablespoons chopped
  parsley, to garnish

1 Preheat the slow cooker if necessary. Spray a large frying pan with a little low-calorie cooking oil spray and place over a high heat until hot. Add the lamb steaks and cook for 4–5 minutes, turning once, until browned on both sides. Transfer to a plate.

2 Add the onion to the frying pan and cook for 4–5 minutes until softened, then add the garlic, lemon and tomatoes. Add the coriander seeds, bay leaf, sweetener, tomato paste and lamb stock, season to taste and bring to the boil.

3 Arrange the potatoes over the base of the slow cooker pot, then place the lamb steaks in a single layer on top. Pour over the hot stock mixture, cover and cook on Low for 9–10 hours until the lamb and potatoes are tender.

4 Add the courgettes, cover again and cook on High for 15–30 minutes until tender. Spoon into shallow bowls, sprinkle with the parsley and serve immediately.

---

for slow-cooked lamb with rosemary

CALORIES PER SERVING 352

Follow the recipe above, adding 3 rosemary sprigs instead of the lemon, coriander seeds and bay leaf. Cook as above, adding the courgettes at the end. Serve garnished with the parsley.

braised trout with warm puy lentils

400 g (13 oz) can Puy lentils, drained

2 tablespoons balsamic vinegar

4 spring onions, chopped

3 tomatoes, chopped

4 thick trout steaks, 150 g (5 oz) each

finely grated rind and juice of ½ lemon

leaves from 2-3 thyme sprigs

large pinch of dried chilli flakes

150 ml (¼ pint) hot fish stock

salt and pepper

50 g (2 oz) rocket leaves, to serve

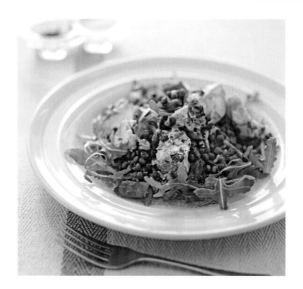

for smoked cod & spinach salad

CALORIES PER SERVING 228

Follow the recipe above, using 100 g (3½ oz) sliced button mushrooms instead of the tomatoes, and 4 thick smoked cod loin steaks, 150 g (5 oz) each, instead of the trout. After cooking, stir 50 g (2 oz) baby spinach leaves into the lentil mixture and serve each portion topped with a poached egg.

1 Preheat the slow cooker if necessary. Place the lentils in the slow cooker pot, then stir in the balsamic vinegar, spring onions and tomatoes.

2 Arrange the trout steaks on top in a single layer, then sprinkle with the lemon rind and juice, thyme leaves and chilli flakes and season to taste. Pour the stock around the trout steaks, then cover and cook on Low for 2½-3 hours or until the trout is cooked through and flakes easily when pressed with a small knife.

3 Divide the rocket leaves between 4 serving plates. Arrange the trout and lentils on top and spoon over a little of the stock. Serve immediately.

slimming cassoulet

low-calorie cooking oil spray

500 g (1 lb) lean pork, diced

75 g (3 oz) chorizo, sliced

1 onion, chopped

3 garlic cloves, finely chopped

1 red pepper, cored, deseeded
    and diced

2 celery sticks, sliced

1 carrot, diced

500 g (1 lb) passata

1 teaspoon dried
    Mediterranean herbs

2 x 375 g (12 oz) cans cannellini
    beans, drained

3 tablespoons fresh
    breadcrumbs

salt and pepper

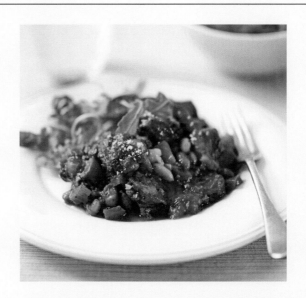

for chicken cassoulet

CALORIES PER SERVING 346

Follow the recipe above, using 500 g (1 lb) boneless, skinless chicken thighs, diced, instead of the pork. Mix the breadcrumbs with 2 tablespoons chopped rosemary and 2 tablespoons chopped parsley, then spoon over the cassoulet and cook as above.

1 Preheat the slow cooker if necessary. Spray a large frying pan with a little low-calorie cooking oil spray and place over a high heat until hot. Add the pork, a few pieces at a time until all the pork is in the pan, and cook for 5 minutes, stirring, until browned. Use a slotted spoon to transfer the pork to the slow cooker pot.

2 Add the chorizo and onion to the frying pan and cook for 4–5 minutes until the onion has softened. Stir in the garlic, red pepper, celery, carrot, passata and herbs. Season to taste and bring to the boil, stirring.

3 Place the beans in the slow cooker pot, pour over the passata mixture and stir well. Level the surface with the back of a spoon, then sprinkle over the breadcrumbs. Cover and cook on Low for 8–10 hours until the pork is tender. Spoon into shallow bowls and serve with salad, if liked.

tangy turkey tagine

low-calorie cooking oil spray

400 g (13 oz) turkey breast, diced

1 onion, chopped

2 garlic cloves, finely chopped

1 tablespoon plain flour

450 ml (¾ pint) chicken stock

2 pinches of saffron strands or 1 teaspoon ground turmeric

5 cm (2 inch) cinnamon stick

finely grated rind of 1 lemon

400 g (13 oz) can chickpeas, drained

25 g (1 oz) sultanas

salt and pepper

TO SERVE

175 g (6 oz) couscous

450 ml (¾ pint) boiling water

4 tablespoons chopped mint or mixed mint and parsley

1 Preheat the slow cooker if necessary. Spray a large frying pan with a little low-calorie cooking oil spray and place over a high heat until hot. Add the turkey, a few pieces at a time until all the turkey is in the pan, and cook for 5 minutes, stirring until golden. Use a slotted spoon to transfer the turkey to a plate.

2 Add the onion to the frying pan and cook for 4–5 minutes until softened. Stir in the garlic and flour, then add the stock and mix well. Add the saffron or turmeric, cinnamon and lemon rind, then the chickpeas and sultanas. Season to taste and bring to the boil, stirring.

3 Pour into the slow cooker pot, add the turkey pieces and press into the liquid. Cover and cook on Low for 8–9 hours until the turkey is tender and cooked through.

4 Meanwhile, place the couscous in a mixing bowl, pour over the boiling water, cover with a plate and leave to soak for 5 minutes until tender. Stir in the chopped herbs, season to taste and fluff up with a fork. Divide the couscous between 4 plates and top with the tagine. Serve with naan, if liked.

for harissa-baked turkey
CALORIES PER SERVING 396

Follow the recipe above, using 300 ml (½ pint) chicken stock and 250 g (8 oz) diced tomatoes instead of 450 ml (¾ pint) chicken stock. Omit the saffron, cinnamon and lemon and add 2 teaspoons harissa paste and 2.5 cm (1 inch) piece of fresh root ginger, chopped, instead. Cook as above and serve with the herby couscous.

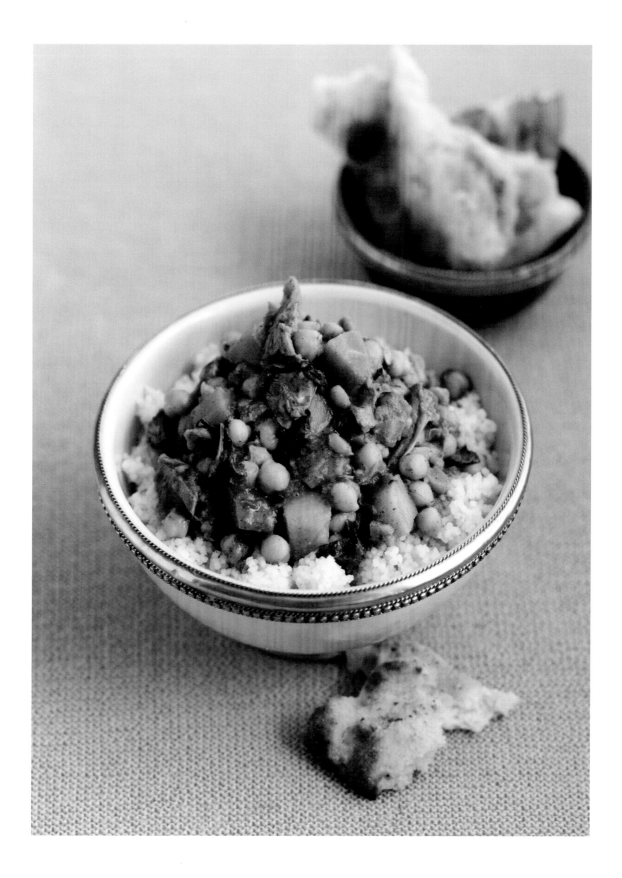

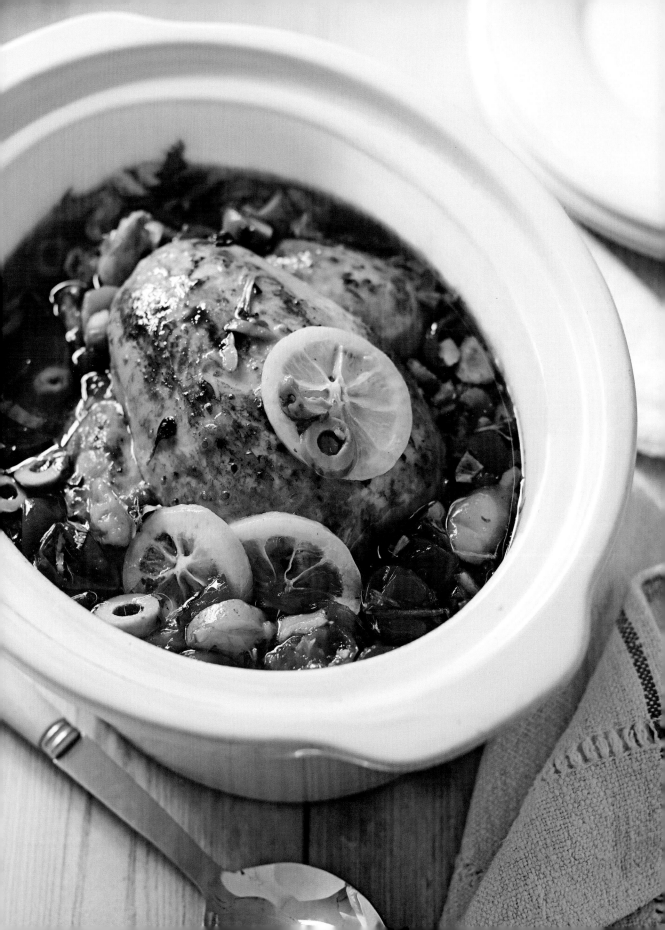

chicken & pepper pot roast

1.35 kg (2 lb 10 oz) oven-ready
  chicken

225 g (7½ oz) baby new
  potatoes, halved

1 red pepper, cored, deseeded
  and diced

1 yellow pepper, cored,
  deseeded and diced

4 garlic cloves, halved

200 g (7 oz) cherry tomatoes,
  halved

½ lemon, sliced

small bunch of basil

300 ml (½ pint) hot
  chicken stock

1 tablespoon tomato purée

3 teaspoons granular
  sweetener

40 g (1½ oz) pitted green
olives in brine, drained and
  halved

salt and pepper

1 Preheat the slow cooker if necessary. Put the chicken into the
slow cooker pot, then tuck the potatoes, peppers, garlic and
tomatoes around it. Season the chicken, then arrange the
lemon slices over the breast. Tear half the basil into pieces and
sprinkle over the chicken and vegetables.

2 Mix the hot stock with the tomato purée and sweetener, then
pour into the slow cooker pot and add the olives. Cover and
cook on High for 5–6 hours or until the chicken is thoroughly
cooked and the meat juices run clear when the thickest parts
of the leg and breast are pierced with a sharp knife.

3 Place the slow cooker pot under a preheated hot grill until the
chicken is golden. Cut the meat off the bones and arrange it in
shallow bowls with the vegetables and stock, garnished with
the remaining basil. If you prefer a thicker sauce, drain the
stock into a small saucepan and boil rapidly to reduce by half.

---

for lemon & tarragon pot-roasted chicken

CALORIES PER SERVING 470

Place the chicken in the slow cooker pot and tuck 225 g (7½ oz)
halved baby new potatoes, 3 chopped carrots, 3 chopped celery
sticks and 2 tarragon sprigs around it. Season the chicken and
cover the breast with ½ sliced lemon. Mix 300 ml (½ pint) hot
chicken stock with 1 tablespoon tomato purée and 3 teaspoons
Dijon mustard and pour over the chicken. Cook as above and
serve garnished with extra tarragon.

pork stew with sweet potatoes

low-calorie cooking oil spray

500 g (1 lb) lean pork, cubed

1 onion, chopped

125 g (4 oz) closed-cap
   mushrooms, sliced

450 ml (¾ pint) chicken stock

2 tablespoons tomato purée

2 tablespoons soy sauce

¼ teaspoon chilli powder

½ teaspoon ground allspice

¼ teaspoon ground cinnamon

1 teaspoon granular sweetener

150 g (5 oz) carrots,
   thinly sliced

2 celery sticks, thickly sliced

375 g (12 oz) sweet potato, cut
   into 2.5 cm (1 inch) chunks

125 g (4 oz) curly kale,
   shredded

1 Preheat the slow cooker if necessary. Spray a large frying pan with a little low-calorie cooking oil spray and place over a high heat until hot. Add the pork, a few pieces at a time until all the pork is in the pan, and cook for 3 minutes, stirring. Add the onion and cook for a further 2–3 minutes until the pork is golden.

2 Stir in the mushrooms, then add the stock, tomato purée and soy sauce. Add the chilli powder, allspice, cinnamon and sweetener, season to taste and bring to the boil, stirring.

3 Place the carrots, celery and sweet potato in the slow cooker pot, then pour over the pork and sauce. Press the meat into the liquid, cover and cook on Low for 8–9 hours until the pork is tender.

4 Stir the stew, then add the kale. Cover again and cook on High for 15 minutes, then spoon into bowls and serve immediately.

for fragrant sausage & sweet potato stew
CALORIES PER SERVING 362

Place 500 g (1 lb) reduced-fat pork sausages under a preheated hot grill until browned but not cooked through. Transfer to the slow cooker pot. Continue with the recipe above, omitting the pork.

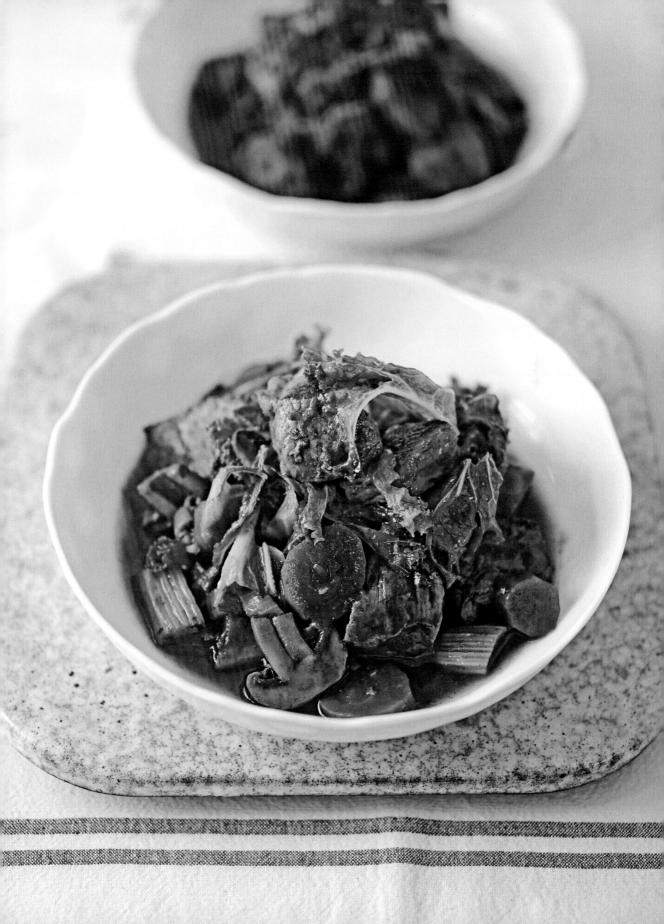

sweet & sour chicken

1 tablespoon sunflower oil

1 kg (2 lb) boneless, skinless
  chicken thighs, cubed

4 spring onions, thickly sliced

2 carrots, halved lengthways
  and thinly sliced

2.5 cm (1 inch) piece of fresh
  root ginger, finely chopped

425 g (14 oz) can pineapple
  chunks in natural juice

300 ml (½ pint) chicken stock

1 tablespoon cornflour

1 tablespoon tomato purée

2 tablespoons caster sugar

2 tablespoons soy sauce

2 tablespoons malt vinegar

225 g (7½ oz) can bamboo
  shoots, drained

125 g (4 oz) bean sprouts

100 g (3½ oz) mangetout,
  thinly sliced

150 g (5 oz) rice, boiled

for lemon chicken

CALORIES PER SERVING 438

Follow the recipe above as far as
the addition of the stock. Mix the
cornflour to a paste with the juice
of 1 lemon, then stir into the pan
with 2 tablespoons dry sherry
and 4 teaspoons caster sugar.
Bring to a boil, stirring, then
transfer to the slow cooker pot
and continue with steps 3 and 4.

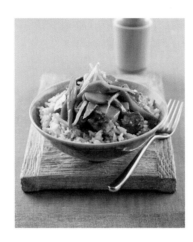

1   Preheat the slow cooker if
    necessary. Heat the oil in a
    large frying pan over a high
    heat, add the chicken and
    cook for 3–4 minutes until
    browned on all sides. Add
    the white spring onion slices
    (reserving the green slices),
    the carrots and ginger and
    cook for 2 minutes.

2   Stir in the pineapple chunks
    and their juice and the
    stock. Put the cornflour,
    tomato purée and sugar in
    a small bowl, then mix in the
    soy sauce and vinegar to
    make a smooth paste. Add to
    the pan and bring to the
    boil, stirring.

3   Transfer the chicken
    mixture to the slow cooker
    pot, add the bamboo
    shoots and press the
    chicken pieces into the
    liquid. Cover and cook on
    Low for 6–8 hours until the
    chicken is cooked through.

4   Add the reserved green
    spring onion slices,
    the bean sprouts and
    mangetout and mix well.
    Cover again and cook for
    15 minutes or until the
    vegetables are just tender.
    Serve with the boiled rice.

cidered gammon hotpot

500 g (1 lb) unsmoked
   gammon joint, trimmed of fat
625 g (1 ¼ lb) baking potatoes,
   cut into 2 cm (¾ inch) chunks
200 g (7 oz) small shallots,
   peeled
3 carrots, thickly sliced
2 celery sticks, thickly sliced
1 large leek, thickly sliced
2 bay leaves
200 ml (7 fl oz) dry cider
200 ml (7 fl oz) hot chicken
   stock
¼ teaspoon cloves
1 teaspoon mustard powder
pepper
3 tablespoons chopped chives,
   to garnish

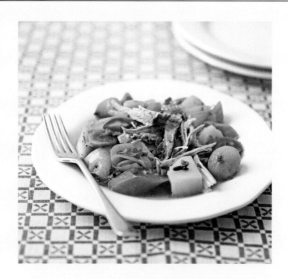

1 Preheat the slow cooker if necessary. Rinse the gammon joint with cold water and place in the slow cooker pot with the potatoes. Arrange the shallots, carrots, celery and leek slices around the gammon, then tuck in the bay leaves.

2 Pour the cider and stock into a saucepan, add the cloves and mustard powder, then season with pepper (gammon joints can be salty so don't be tempted to add salt). Bring to the boil, then pour around the gammon. Cover and cook on High for 6-7 hours until the gammon is cooked through.

3 Cut the gammon into pieces and serve in shallow bowls with the vegetables and stock, garnished with chopped chives.

for gammon in cola

CALORIES PER SERVING 376

Follow the recipe above, using 450 ml (¾ pint) diet cola instead of the cider and stock and omitting the potatoes. Serve with 625 g (1¼ lb) boiled baby new potatoes and 150 g (5 oz) steamed green beans.

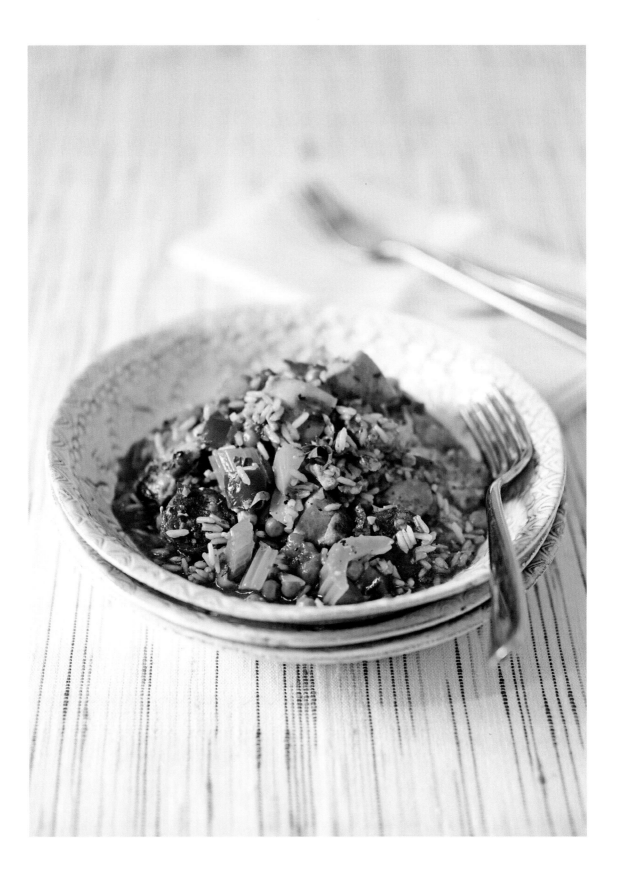

simple paella

low-calorie cooking oil spray

500 g (1 lb) boneless, skinless
chicken thighs, cubed

1 onion, chopped

60 g (2¼ oz) chorizo, sliced

2 garlic cloves, finely chopped

1 red pepper, cored, deseeded
and diced

1 orange pepper, cored,
deseeded and diced

2 celery sticks, diced

2 pinches of saffron threads

½ teaspoon dried
Mediterranean herbs

750 ml (1¼ pints) hot chicken
stock

175 g (6 oz) long-grain
brown rice

125 g (4 oz) frozen peas

salt and pepper

2 tablespoons chopped
parsley, to garnish

1 Preheat the slow cooker if necessary. Spray a large frying pan
with a little low-calorie cooking oil spray and place over a high
heat until hot. Add the chicken, a few pieces at a time until all
the chicken is in the pan, and cook for 5 minutes, stirring, until
browned. Use a slotted spoon to transfer the chicken to the
slow cooker pot.

2 Add the onion, chorizo and garlic to the frying pan and cook
for 3–4 minutes, stirring until the onion is beginning to colour.
Add the peppers and celery, stir well, then transfer to the slow
cooker pot. Mix the saffron and dried herbs with the hot stock,
season to taste, then pour into the slow cooker pot and stir
well. Cover and cook on High for 3–4 hours.

3 Place the rice in a sieve and rinse under cold running water,
then stir into the chicken mixture. Cover again and cook
for 1½–1¾ hours until the rice is tender. Stir in the peas and
continue cooking for 15 minutes. Serve garnished with
chopped parsley.

---

for seafood paella

CALORIES PER SERVING 385

Follow the recipe above to cook the paella, omitting the
chicken. Defrost a 400 g (13 oz) packet of frozen mixed seafood
and pat dry on kitchen paper. Spray a large frying pan with a
little low-calorie cooking oil spray and place over a high heat
until hot. Add the seafood and fry for 4–5 minutes until piping
hot. Stir into the finished paella and garnish with the parsley.

pork puttanesca

low-calorie cooking oil spray

625 g (1¼ lb) lean pork, diced

1 onion, chopped

2 garlic cloves, finely chopped

400 g (13 oz) can chopped
   tomatoes

4 teaspoons sherry vinegar

15 g (½ oz) basil, roughly torn,
   plus extra to garnish

1 tablespoon capers in brine,
   drained and chopped

50 g (2 oz) pitted olives,
   chopped

salt and pepper

chopped parsley, to garnish

175 g (6 oz) spaghetti, boiled

1 Preheat the slow cooker if necessary. Spray a large frying pan with a little low-calorie cooking oil spray and place over a high heat until hot. Add the pork, a few pieces at a time until all the pork is in the pan, and cook for 5 minutes, stirring, until browned. Use a slotted spoon to transfer the pork to a plate.

2 Add a little more low-calorie cooking oil spray to the frying pan, then add the onion and cook for 4–5 minutes, stirring, until just beginning to brown. Add the garlic, tomatoes, vinegar and basil and bring to the boil, stirring.

3 Mix the capers and olives together and add half to the sauce, reserving the rest for garnish.

4 Transfer the pork to the slow cooker pot, then pour over the sauce. Cover and cook on High for 7–8 hours until the pork is tender. Stir, then sprinkle with the reserved capers and olives, some extra basil and a little chopped parsley. Serve with the cooked spaghetti.

for garlic & lemon pork

CALORIES PER SERVING 436

Follow the recipe above, using 2 tablespoons chopped parsley mixed with the grated rind of 1 lemon and 2 finely chopped garlic cloves instead of the capers and olives. Serve with 225 g (7½ oz) rice, boiled with a few strands of saffron.

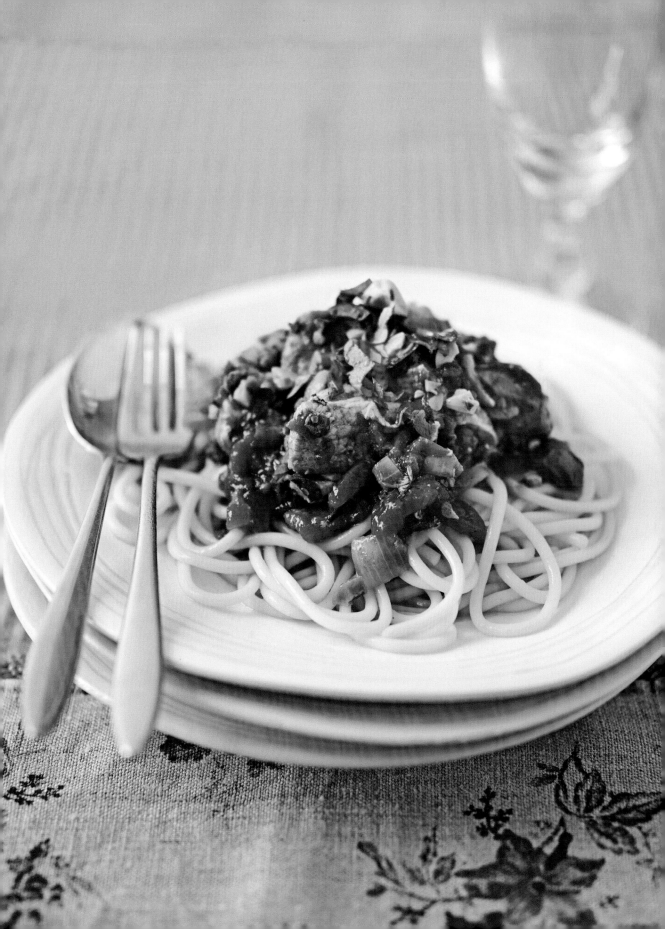

beef bourguignon

low-calorie cooking oil spray

625 g (1¼ lb) stewing beef,
   trimmed of fat and cubed

100 g (3½ oz) bacon, diced

300 g (10 oz) small shallots,
   peeled

3 garlic cloves, finely chopped

1 tablespoon plain flour

150 ml (¼ pint) red wine

300 ml (½ pint) beef stock

1 tablespoon tomato purée

small bunch of mixed herbs or
   a dried bouquet garni

salt and pepper

chopped parsley, to garnish

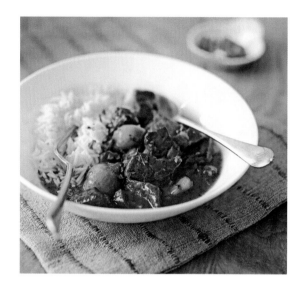

1   Preheat the slow cooker if necessary. Spray a large frying pan with a little low-calorie cooking oil spray and place over a high heat until hot. Add the beef, a few pieces at a time until all the beef is in the pan, and cook for 5 minutes, stirring, until browned. Use a slotted spoon to transfer the beef to the slow cooker pot.

2   Add the bacon and shallots to the frying pan and cook over a medium heat for 2–3 minutes until the bacon is just beginning to brown. Stir in the garlic and flour, then add the wine, stock, tomato purée and herbs. Season to taste and bring to the boil, stirring.

3   Pour the sauce over the beef, cover and cook on Low for 10–11 hours until the beef is tender. Stir, garnish with chopped parsley and serve with rice, if liked.

for beef goulash

CALORIES PER SERVING 319

Follow the recipe above, adding 2 teaspoons mild paprika, 1 teaspoon caraway seeds, ¼ teaspoon ground cinnamon and ¼ teaspoon ground allspice instead of the herbs.

chicken cacciatore

low-calorie cooking oil spray

500 g (1 lb) boneless, skinless chicken
   thighs, cubed

1 onion, chopped

2 garlic cloves, finely chopped

1 red pepper, cored, deseeded and diced

1 orange pepper, cored, deseeded and
   diced

2 celery sticks, diced

150 ml (¼ pint) chicken stock

400 g (13 oz) can chopped tomatoes

1 tablespoon tomato purée

1 tablespoon balsamic vinegar

leaves from 2 rosemary sprigs, chopped

salt and pepper

2 tablespoons chopped parsley,
   to garnish

200 g (7 oz) dried tagliatelle, to serve

for potato-topped cacciatore

CALORIES PER SERVING 403

Follow the recipe above and place all the
ingredients in the slow cooker pot. Thinly
slice 625 g (1¼ lb) potatoes and arrange
them on top of the chicken mixture,
overlapping. Press the potatoes down
into the liquid, then cover and cook on
High for 5–6 hours until the potatoes and
chicken are cooked through. Spray the
potatoes with a little extra low-calorie
cooking oil spray, then place the slow
cooker pot under a hot grill until the
potatoes are golden, if liked.

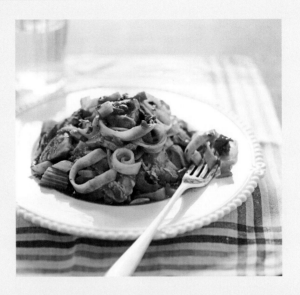

1 Preheat the slow cooker if necessary. Spray a large frying
   pan with a little low-calorie cooking oil spray and place
   over a high heat until hot. Add the chicken, a few pieces
   at a time until all the chicken is in the pan, and cook for
   3–4 minutes, stirring, until just beginning to brown.
   Add the onion and continue to cook until the chicken is
   golden and the onion has softened.

2 Stir in the garlic, peppers and celery, then add the
   stock, tomatoes, tomato purée, balsamic vinegar and
   rosemary. Season generously and bring to the boil,
   stirring. Transfer to the slow cooker pot, cover and cook
   on Low for 8–9 hours until the chicken is tender and
   cooked through.

3 Meanwhile, cook the tagliatelle in a saucepan of lightly
   salted boiling water according to packet instructions
   until tender. Drain, then toss with the chicken mixture
   and serve garnished with parsley.

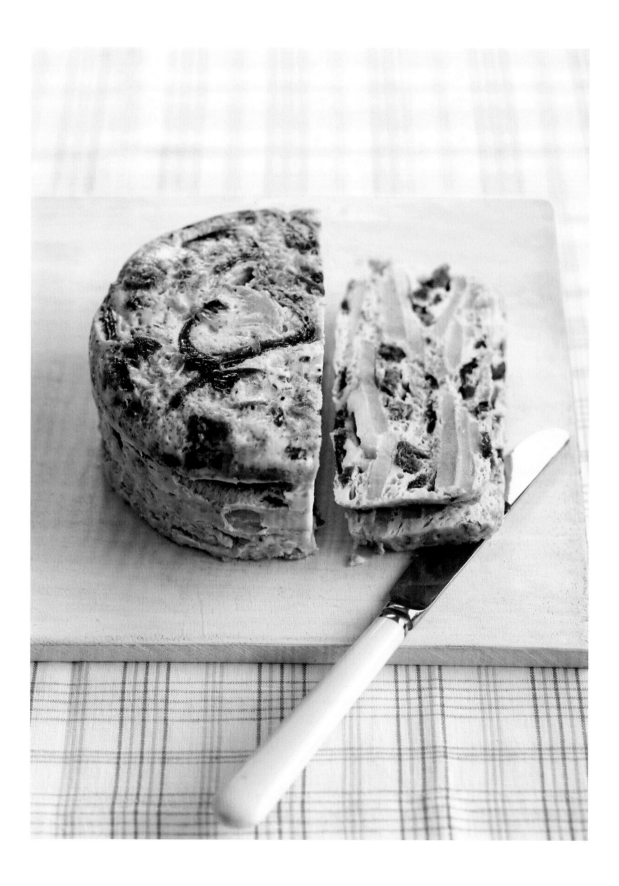

red pepper & chorizo tortilla

1 tablespoon olive oil, plus
   extra for greasing
1 small onion, chopped
75 g (3 oz) chorizo, diced
6 eggs
150 ml (¼ pint) milk
100 g (3½ oz) roasted red
   peppers from a jar, sliced
250 g (8 oz) cooked potatoes,
   sliced
salt and pepper

1 Preheat the slow cooker if necessary. Lightly oil a 1.2 litre (2 pint) ovenproof soufflé dish and line the base with non-stick baking paper. Heat the oil in a small frying pan over a medium heat, add the onion and chorizo and cook for 4–5 minutes until the onion has softened.

2 Beat the eggs and milk together in a mixing bowl and season to taste. Add the onion and chorizo, red pepper and potatoes and toss together.

3 Tip the mixture into the oiled dish, cover the top with foil and put in the slow cooker pot. Pour boiling water into the slow cooker pot to come halfway up the sides of the dish, cover and cook on High for 2–2½ hours until the egg mixture has just set in the centre.

4 Loosen the edges of the tortilla with a round-bladed knife, turn it out on to a plate and peel off the lining paper. Cut into slices and serve hot or cold, with salad if liked.

for cheesy bacon & rosemary tortilla
CALORIES PER SERVING 282

Follow the recipe above, using 75 g (3 oz) diced smoked streaky bacon instead of the chorizo. Beat the eggs and milk in a bowl with the chopped leaves from 2 small rosemary sprigs, 4 tablespoons freshly grated Parmesan or Cheddar cheese and 75 g (3 oz) sliced button mushrooms. Season to taste and continue as above.

salmon bourride

low-calorie cooking oil spray

1 onion, chopped

2 garlic cloves, finely chopped

½ red pepper, cored, deseeded
and very thinly sliced

½ orange pepper, cored,
deseeded and very
thinly sliced

400 g (13 oz) can chopped
tomatoes

150 ml (¼ pint) vegetable stock

1 teaspoon granular sweetener

1 teaspoon cornflour

400 g (13 oz) can artichoke
hearts, drained

4 salmon steaks, 140 g
(4½ oz) each

finely grated rind of 1 lemon

½ teaspoon dried
Mediterranean herbs

salt and pepper

200 g (7 oz) steamed green
beans, to serve

1 Preheat the slow cooker if necessary. Spray a large frying pan with a little low-calorie cooking oil spray and place over a high heat until hot. Add the onion, garlic and peppers and cook for 4–5 minutes until softened.

2 Stir in the tomatoes, stock and sweetener. Mix the cornflour to a smooth paste with a little cold water and stir into the pan. Season to taste and bring to the boil, stirring.

3 Transfer the mixture into the slow cooker pot, stir in the artichoke hearts, then arrange the salmon steaks in a single layer on top, pressing them down into the liquid. Sprinkle the lemon rind and herbs over the salmon and season lightly.

4 Cover and cook on Low for 3–3½ hours until the salmon steaks are cooked and flake easily when pressed with a small knife. Spoon into shallow bowls and serve with the steamed green beans.

---

for squid bourride

CALORIES PER SERVING 205

Rinse 625 g (1¼ lb) prepared squid and take the tentacles out of the tubes. Slice the squid tubes and drain well. Follow the recipe above, using the sliced squid tubes instead of the salmon and cooking on Low for 4–5 hours. Add the squid tentacles and continue cooking for 30 minutes until tender, then serve with the steamed green beans.

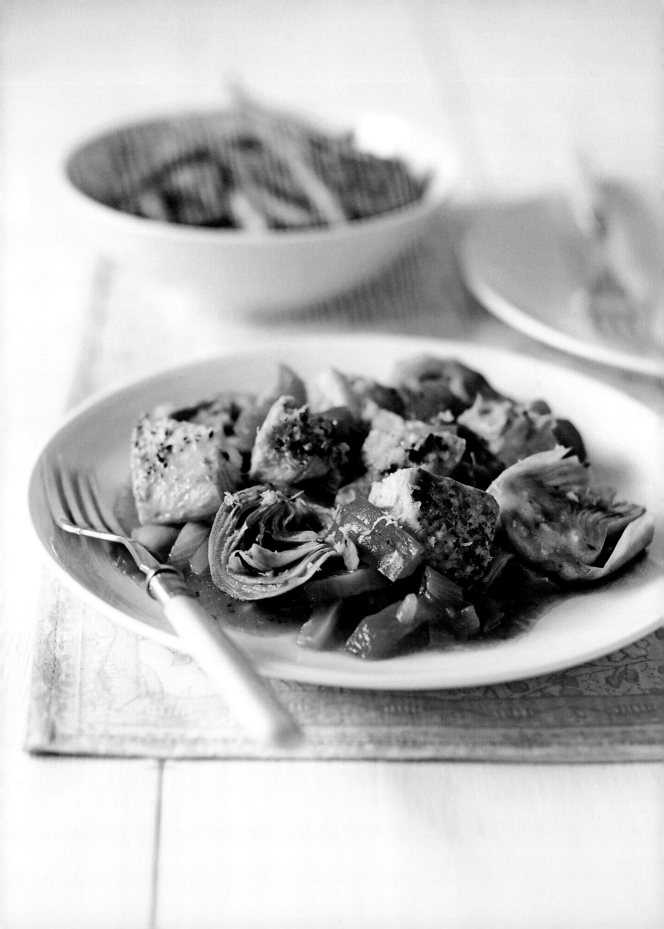

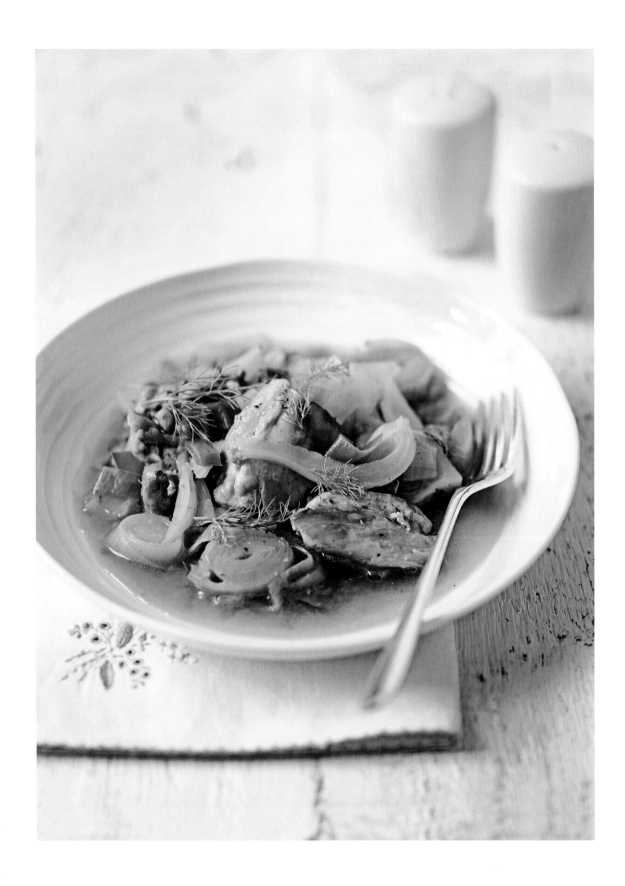

tangy chicken fennel & leek braise

low-calorie cooking oil spray

625 g (1¼ lb) boneless, skinless
chicken thighs, halved

1 fennel bulb, cored and sliced,
green fronds reserved

2 leeks, thinly sliced

350 ml (12 fl oz) chicken stock

finely grated rind and juice of
½ orange

2 teaspoons cornflour

salt and pepper

1 Preheat the slow cooker if necessary. Spray a large frying pan with a little low-calorie cooking oil spray and place over a high heat until hot. Add the chicken and cook for 3–4 minutes, turning once, until browned on both sides. Use a slotted spoon to transfer to a plate.

2 Add the fennel and white leek slices to the frying pan, reserving the green slices. Cook for 2–3 minutes until just beginning to soften, then add the stock, and orange rind and juice. Mix the cornflour to a smooth paste with a little cold water and stir into the pan. Season to taste and bring to the boil, stirring.

3 Transfer the mixture to the slow cooker pot, arrange the chicken pieces on top in a single layer and press into the liquid. Cover and cook on Low for 8–9 hours until the chicken is cooked through.

4 Add the reserved green leek slices, stir into the sauce, cover again and cook for 30 minutes. Serve garnished with the reserved fennel fronds.

for braised mustard chicken & leeks
CALORIES PER SERVING 323

Follow the recipe above, using 75 g (3 oz) diced lean back bacon instead of the fennel. Use 1 teaspoon Dijon mustard instead of the orange rind and juice and cook as above. Garnish with chopped parsley.

lamb steaks with cumberland sauce

1 tablespoon sunflower oil

800 g (1 lb 9 oz) lamb rump
   steaks, trimmed of fat

1 onion, sliced

2 teaspoons plain flour

125 ml (4 fl oz) red wine

125 ml (4 fl oz) lamb stock

finely shredded rind and juice
   of 1 orange

finely shredded rind and juice
   of 1 lemon

2.5 cm (1 inch) piece of fresh
   root ginger, finely chopped

1 tablespoon tomato purée

1 tablespoon redcurrant jelly

1 tablespoon granular
   sweetener

salt and pepper

750 g (1½ lb) celeriac, diced, to
   serve

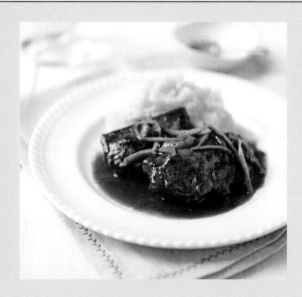

for lamb steaks with cranberry sauce

CALORIES PER SERVING 444

Follow the recipe above, using
25 g (1 oz) dried cranberries
and 1 tablespoon cranberry
sauce instead of the ginger and
redcurrant jelly. Cook and serve
as above.

1 Preheat the slow cooker if necessary. Heat the oil in a large
frying pan over a high heat until hot. Add the lamb and cook
for 2–3 minutes, turning once, until browned on both sides.
Use a slotted spoon to transfer the lamb to the slow
cooker pot.

2 Add the onion to the pan and cook for 4–5 minutes over a
medium heat, stirring until softened. Stir in the flour, then add
the wine, stock, half the orange and lemon rind, the orange
and lemon juice, the ginger, tomato purée, redcurrant jelly
and sweetener. Season to taste and bring to the boil, stirring.
Pour the mixture over the lamb, cover and cook on Low for
8–10 hours.

3 Cook the celeriac in a saucepan of lightly salted boiling
water for 10–15 minutes until tender. Mash with a little of the
cooking water until smooth and season to taste. Serve with
the lamb in bowls, garnished with the remaining orange and
lemon rind.

beery barley beef

1 tablespoon sunflower oil
625 g (1¼ lb) lean stewing beef,
    cubed
1 onion, chopped
1 tablespoon plain flour
250 g (8 oz) carrots, diced
250 g (8 oz) parsnips or
    potatoes, diced
300 ml (½ pint) light ale
750 ml (1¼ pint) beef stock
small bunch of mixed herbs or
    dried bouquet garni
100 g (3½ oz) pearl barley
salt and pepper

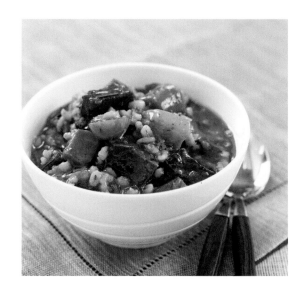

1 Preheat the slow cooker if necessary. Heat the oil in a frying
pan, add the beef a few pieces at a time until it is all in
the pan, then fry over a high heat, stirring, until browned.
Remove the beef with a slotted spoon and transfer to the
slow cooker pot.

2 Add the onion to the frying pan and fry, stirring, for
5 minutes or until lightly browned. Mix in the flour, then
add the root vegetables and beer and bring to the boil,
stirring. Pour into the slow cooker pot.

for herb croutons to accompany the beef

CALORIES PER SERVING 433

Beat 2 tablespoons chopped
parsley, 2 tablespoons chopped
chives and 1 tablespoon chopped
tarragon and a little black pepper
into 75 g (3 oz) soft butter. Thickly
slice ½ French stick, toast lightly
on both sides, then spread with
the herb butter.

3 Add the stock to the frying pan with the herbs and a little
salt and pepper, bring to the boil, then pour into the slow
cooker pot. Add the pearl barley, cover with the lid and cook
on low for 9–10 hours until the beef is tender. Serve with
herb croutons, if liked.

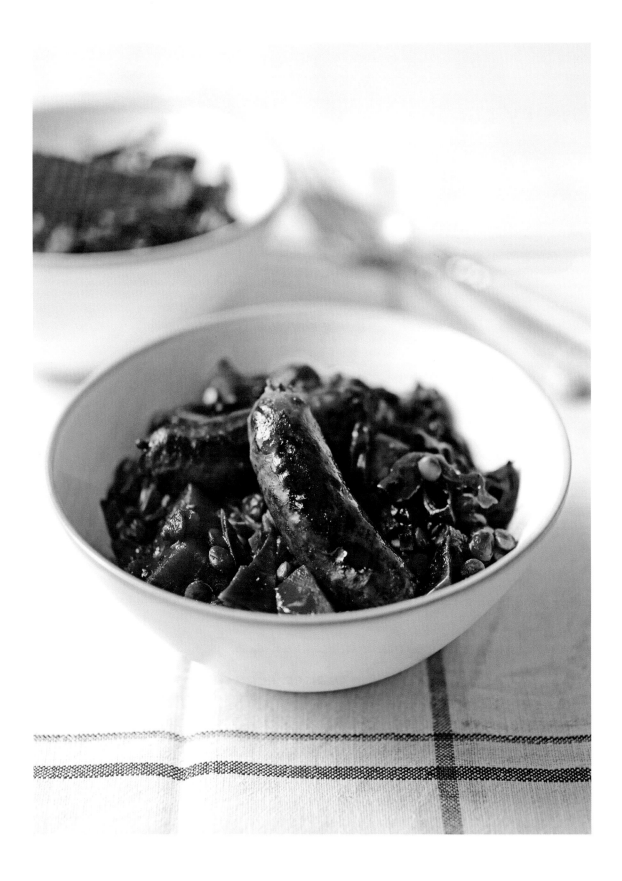

venison sausages with red cabbage

8 venison sausages, 525 g
 (1 lb 1 oz) in total
low-calorie cooking oil spray
1 onion, chopped
150 ml (¼ pint) red wine
600 ml (1 pint) beef stock
2 tablespoons cranberry sauce
1 tablespoon tomato purée
2 bay leaves
300 g (10 oz) potatoes, cut
 into 2.5 cm (1 inch) chunks
2 carrots, cut into 2 cm
 (¾ inch) chunks
250 g (8 oz) tomatoes,
 roughly chopped
250 g (8 oz) red cabbage,
 finely shredded
125 g (4 oz) dried green lentils
salt and pepper

1   Preheat the slow cooker if necessary. Cook the sausages under a preheated medium grill for 5 minutes, turning until browned but not cooked through.

2   Meanwhile, spray a large frying pan with a little low-calorie cooking oil spray and place over a medium heat until hot. Add the onion and cook for 4–5 minutes until just softened. Add the red wine, stock, cranberry sauce, tomato purée and bay leaves, then season to taste and bring to the boil, stirring.

3   Place the potatoes and carrots in the slow cooker pot with the tomatoes, red cabbage and lentils on top. Pour over the hot wine mixture, then add the sausages and press down into the liquid. Cover and cook on High for 5–6 hours until the sausages and potatoes are cooked through and the lentils are tender. Serve in shallow bowls.

for braised lamb shanks with red cabbage

CALORIES PER SERVING 335

Omit the venison sausages and brown 4 small lamb shanks, 750 g (1½ lb) in total, in a little low-calorie cooking oil spray in a frying pan, then continue with the recipe above.

fragrant spiced chicken

1.5 kg (3 lb) oven-ready chicken

1 onion, chopped

200 g (7 oz) carrots, sliced

7.5 cm (3 inch) piece of fresh
    root ginger, sliced

2 garlic cloves, sliced

1 large mild red chilli, halved

3 large star anise

4 tablespoons soy sauce

4 tablespoons rice vinegar

1 tablespoon light muscovado
    sugar

900 ml (1½ pints) boiling water

small bunch of fresh coriander

75 g (3 oz) mangetout,
    thickly sliced

150 g (5 oz) pak choi,
    thickly sliced

salt and pepper

200 g (7 oz) dried egg noodles,
    to serve

1 Preheat the slow cooker if necessary. Place chicken, breast side down, in the slow cooker pot. Add the onion, carrots, ginger, garlic, chilli and star anise and spoon over the soy sauce, vinegar and sugar. Pour over the boiling water.

2 Add the coriander stems, reserving the leaves, and season to taste. Cover cook on High for 5–6 hours or until the chicken is thoroughly cooked and the meat juices run clear when the thickest parts of the leg and breast are pierced with a sharp knife.

3 Transfer the chicken to a chopping board and keep warm. Add the mangetout and pak choi to the pot, cover again and cook for 5–10 minutes or until just wilted. Meanwhile, cook the noodles in a saucepan of lightly salted boiling water according to packet instructions, drain well and divide between 4 bowls.

4 Carve the chicken into bite-sized pieces and arrange on top of the noodles with the reserved coriander leaves, then ladle over the hot broth and serve immediately.

for spiced chicken with pesto

CALORIES PER SERVING 454

Put the chicken into the pot with 1 chopped onion, 200 g (7 oz) sliced carrots, 2 sliced garlic cloves, 1 sliced fennel bulb and 1 sliced lemon. Pour over the boiling water as above and replace the coriander with a small bunch of basil. Use 3 chopped tomatoes, 150 g (5 oz) chopped purple sprouting broccoli and 2 tablespoons pesto sauce instead of the mangetout and pak choi. Cook 250 g (8 oz) fresh tagliatelle according to packet instructions to serve with the chicken.

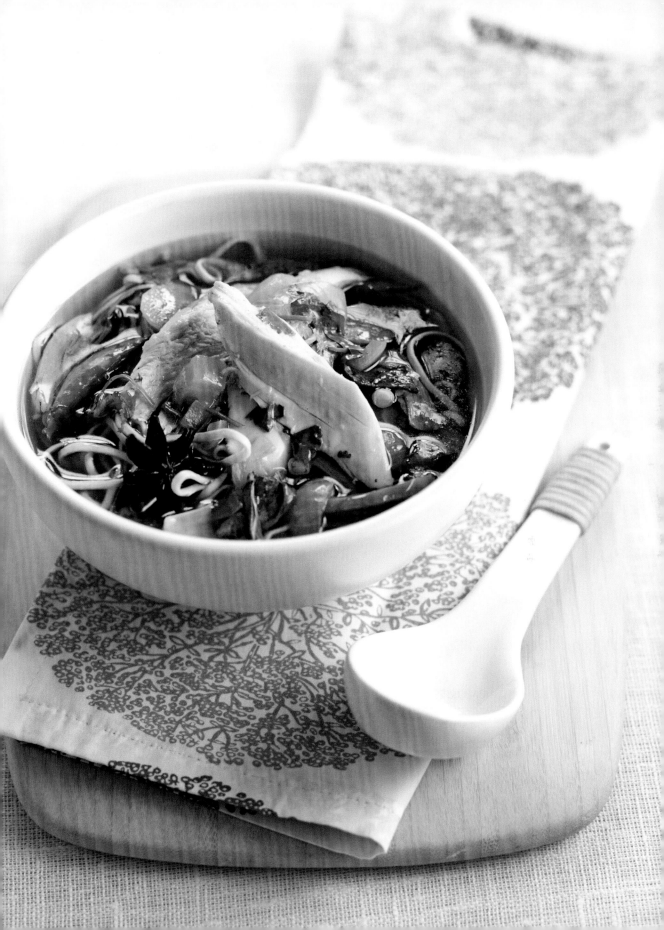

turkey with cranberries & pumpkin

low-calorie cooking oil spray

500 g (1 lb) turkey breast, diced

1 onion, chopped

2 teaspoons plain flour

300 ml (½ pint) chicken stock

juice of 1 large orange

½ teaspoon ground mixed spice

30 g (1¼ oz) dried cranberries

500 g (1 lb) peeled pumpkin, cut into 2.5 cm (1 inch) cubes

salt and pepper

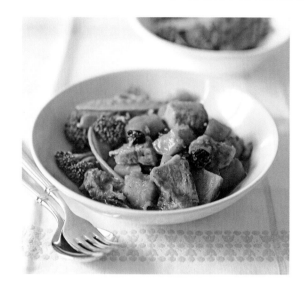

1 Preheat the slow cooker if necessary. Spray a large frying pan with a little low-calorie cooking oil spray and place over a high heat until hot. Add the turkey, a few pieces at a time until all the turkey is in the pan. Add the onion and cook for 5 minutes, stirring and turning the turkey pieces until golden.

2 Sprinkle in the flour and stir well. Add the stock, orange juice, mixed spice and cranberries and season to taste. Bring to the boil, stirring.

3 Place the pumpkin in the slow cooker pot and pour the turkey mixture on top, pushing the turkey pieces into the liquid. Cover and cook on Low for 6–8 hours until the turkey is cooked through. Spoon into shallow dishes and serve with steamed green beans and broccoli, if liked.

for turkey curry with sultanas & pumpkin

CALORIES PER SERVING 279

Follow the recipe above but omit the mixed spice and cranberries and add 3 teaspoons medium-hot curry powder and 25 g (1 oz) sultanas instead.

smoked mackerel rice

1 tablespoon sunflower oil

1 onion, chopped

1 teaspoon ground turmeric

2 tablespoons mango chutney

about 750 ml (1¼ pints)
vegetable stock

1 bay leaf

150 g (5 oz) easy-cook brown
rice

200 g (7 oz) smoked mackerel
fillets, skinned

100 g (3½ oz) frozen peas

25 g (1 oz) watercress or rocket
leaves

4 hard-boiled eggs, cut into
wedges

salt and pepper

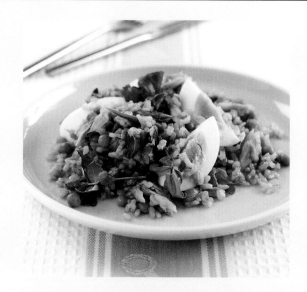

for smoked haddock rice with cardamom

CALORIES PER SERVING 418

Follow the recipe above,
increasing the amount of rice to
175 g (6 oz) and using 4 crushed
cardamom pods with their black
seeds instead of the chutney.
Replace the smoked mackerel
with 400 g (13 oz) skinned
smoked haddock fillet, cut into
2 pieces. Continue as above,
omitting the rocket or watercress.
Drizzle with 4 tablespoons double
cream before serving.

1   Preheat the slow cooker if necessary. Heat the oil in a large
frying pan over a medium heat, add the onion and cook,
stirring, for 5 minutes until softened. Add the turmeric,
chutney, stock and bay leaf, season to taste and bring to
the boil.

2   Pour into the slow cooker pot and add the rice. Arrange the
smoked mackerel in the pot in a single layer, cover and cook
on Low for 3–4 hours until the rice is tender and has absorbed
almost all the stock.

3   Stir in the peas, breaking up the fish into chunky pieces. Add a
little extra hot stock if the rice is very dry, cover again and cook
for 15 minutes. Stir in the watercress or rocket, spoon on to
plates and top with the egg wedges.

balsamic beef hotpot

low-calorie cooking oil spray

600 g (1 lb) lean stewing beef,
trimmed of fat and cubed

1 onion, chopped

250 g (8 oz) swede, cut into
2 cm (¾ inch) cubes

300 g (10 oz) carrots, sliced

150 g (5 oz) mushrooms, sliced

2 teaspoons plain flour

450 ml (¾ pint) beef stock

2 tablespoons balsamic vinegar

1 teaspoon mustard powder

500 g (1 lb) potatoes, sliced

salt and pepper

1 tablespoon chopped parsley,
to garnish

TO SERVE

200 g (7 oz) broccoli florets,
steamed

200 g (7 oz) sugar snap peas,
steamed

1 Preheat the slow cooker if necessary. Spray a large frying pan with a little low-calorie cooking oil spray and place over a high heat until hot. Add the beef, a few pieces at a time until all the beef is in the pan, and cook for 5 minutes, stirring, until browned. Use a slotted spoon to transfer the beef to the slow cooker pot.

2 Add a little more low-calorie cooking oil spray to the pan, add the onion and cook for 4–5 minutes until beginning to brown. Add the swede, carrots and mushrooms and cook for 2 minutes. Add the flour and stir well.

3 Stir in the stock, vinegar and mustard, season to taste and bring to the boil. Pour over the beef in the slow cooker pot. Arrange the potato slices on top, slightly overlapping. Season lightly, then press the potatoes into the stock.

4 Cover and cook on High for 7–8 hours until the potatoes and beef are tender. Spray the potatoes with a little extra low-calorie cooking oil spray, then place the slow cooker pot under a preheated hot grill until the potatoes are golden. Sprinkle with the parsley and serve with the steamed vegetables.

---

for mustard beef hotpot

CALORIES PER SERVING 409

Follow the recipe above, using 1 tablespoon wholegrain mustard in place of the balsamic vinegar and mustard powder.

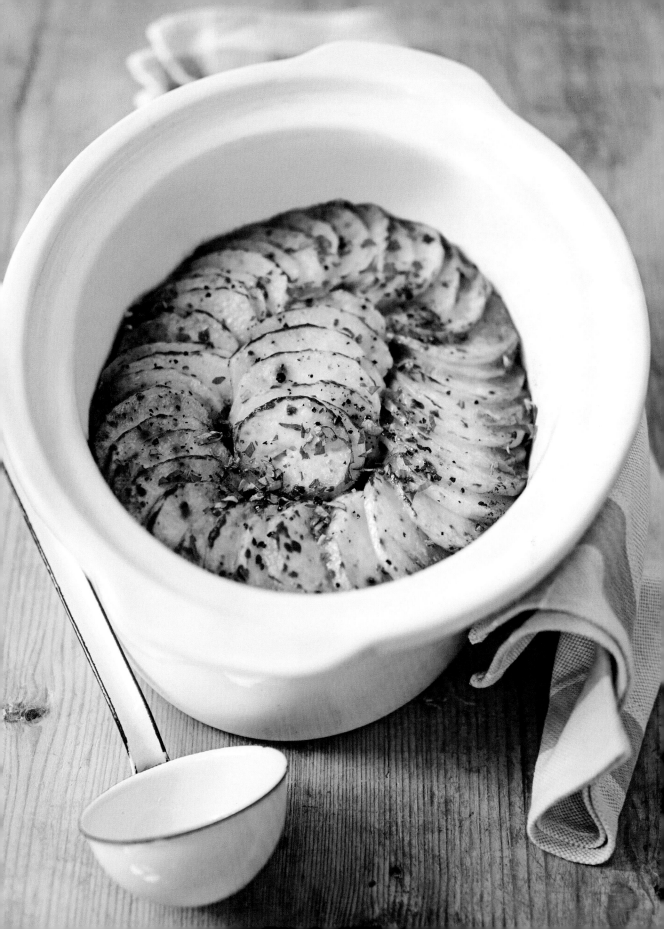

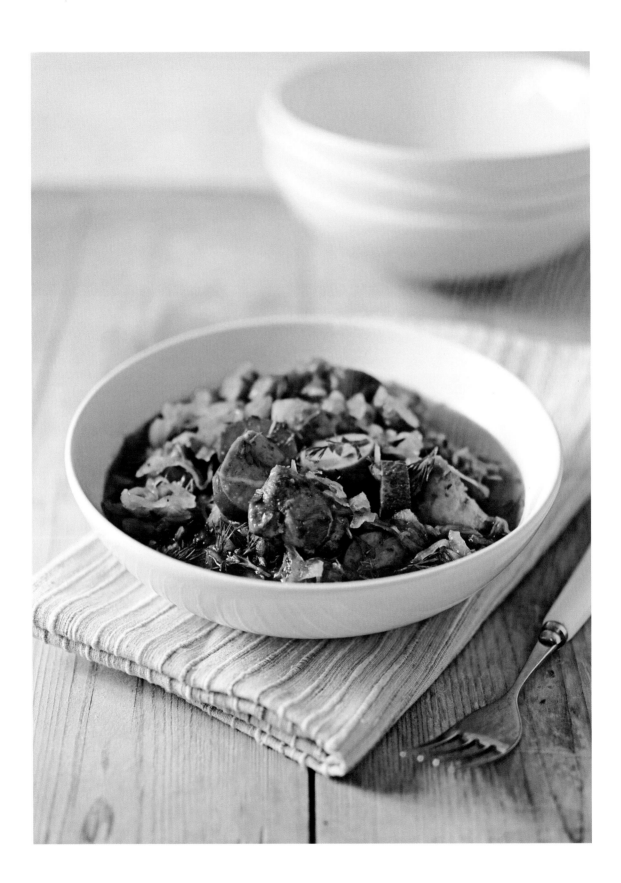

smoked sausage stew

low-calorie cooking oil spray

325 g (11 oz) boneless, skinless chicken thighs, cubed

1 onion, chopped

2 teaspoons mild paprika

1 teaspoon caraway seeds

1 dessert apple, quartered, cored and thinly sliced

250 g (8 oz) tomatoes, diced

1 tablespoon granular sweetener

400 g (13 oz) sauerkraut, drained

200 g (7 oz) smoked pork sausage, sliced

100 g (3½ oz) gherkins, sliced

450 ml (¾ pint) hot chicken stock

salt and pepper

TO GARNISH

3 tablespoons chopped dill

3 tablespoons chopped parsley

1 Preheat the slow cooker if necessary. Spray a large frying pan with a little low-calorie cooking oil spray and place over a high heat until hot. Add the chicken, a few pieces at a time until all the chicken is in the pan, then add the onion and cook for 5 minutes, stirring, until the chicken is golden.

2 Add the paprika, caraway, apple, tomatoes and sweetener to the pan and heat through. Place the sauerkraut in the slow cooker pot and pour the chicken mixture on top, then add the sliced sausage and gherkins.

3 Pour over the hot stock and season to taste. Stir well, cover and cook on Low for 8-10 hours until the chicken is cooked through. Serve in bowls, garnished with chopped dill and parsley.

for chilli pork stew
CALORIES PER SERVING 251

Follow the recipe above, using 500 g (1 lb) diced lean pork instead of the chicken. Use 1 teaspoon mild paprika and 1 teaspoon smoked hot paprika or chilli powder instead of 2 teaspoons mild paprika, and continue with the recipe, omitting the smoked sausage.

turkey tagine

1 turkey drumstick, 700 g
   (1 lb 6 oz)
1 tablespoon olive oil
1 onion, chopped
2 garlic cloves, finely chopped
2.5 cm (1 inch) piece of fresh
   root ginger, finely chopped
2 tablespoons plain flour
1 teaspoon ground turmeric
1 teaspoon ground cinnamon
1 teaspoon ground coriander
½ teaspoon cumin seeds
600 ml (1 pint) hot chicken
   stock
400 g (13 oz) can chickpeas,
   drained
200 g (7 oz) parsnips, diced
200 g (7 oz) carrots, diced
small bunch of fresh coriander,
   roughly chopped
salt and pepper

for chillied chicken tagine

CALORIES PER SERVING 401

Follow the recipe above, using
4 skinless chicken thigh and
drumstick joints instead of the
turkey and adding ½ teaspoon
smoked hot paprika with the
other spices. Cook on High
for 5-6 hours.

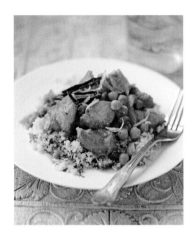

1 Check that the turkey
drumstick will fit into the
slow cooker pot before
you begin, cutting off the
knuckle end if necessary
with a large knife, after
hitting it with a rolling pin
or hammer. Preheat the
slow cooker if necessary.

2 Heat the oil in a frying
pan over a high heat, add
the drumstick and cook,
turning, until golden-
brown all over. Transfer
to the slow cooker pot.
Add the onion to the pan
and cook over a medium
heat for 5 minutes until
softened. Stir in the garlic,
ginger and flour, then mix
in the spices. Gradually
stir in the stock, season to
taste and bring to the boil.

3 Pour the onion mixture
over the turkey. Add the
chickpeas and vegetables
to the pot and press into
the liquid. Cover and cook
on High for 6-7 hours or
until the meat is tender
and almost falling off
the bone.

4 Take the turkey meat off
the bone, discarding the
skin and tendons. Cut it
into bite-sized pieces and
return them to the slow
cooker pot. Stir in the
chopped coriander and
serve with couscous,
if liked.

warming lamb pot roast

low-calorie cooking oil spray
875 g (1¾ lb) leg of lamb on
   the bone
1 leek, thickly sliced
2 teaspoons plain flour
450 ml (¾ pint) lamb stock
1 tablespoon redcurrant jelly
15 g (½ oz) mint leaves,
   chopped, plus extra
   to garnish
200 g (7 oz) celeriac, cut into
   2 cm (¾ inch) cubes
200 g (7 oz) swede, cut into
   2 cm (¾ inch) cubes
300 g (10 oz) baby Chantenay
   carrots, halved lengthways
salt and pepper

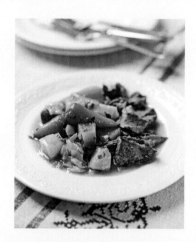

for lamb pot roast with flageolet beans

CALORIES PER SERVING 459

Follow the recipe above, adding a 400 g (13 oz) can of flageolet beans, drained, 2 rosemary sprigs and 2 finely chopped garlic cloves instead of the mint, swede and celeriac.

1   Preheat the slow cooker if necessary. Spray a large frying pan with low-calorie cooking oil spray and place over high heat until hot. Season the lamb and seal in the pan for 5–10 minutes, turning until browned on all sides. Transfer to the slow cooker pot.

2   Add the white leek slices (keeping the green slices) to the pan with a little extra low-calorie cooking oil spray, cook for 2–3 minutes, add in the flour and stir well. Add the stock, jelly and mint, then bring to the boil, stirring.

3   Arrange the celeriac, swede and carrots around the lamb, then pour over the leeks and stock. Cover and cook on High for 5–6 hours until the lamb starts to fall off the bone and the vegetables are tender, adding the reserved green leek slices for the last 15 minutes of cooking.

4   Serve the lamb in shallow bowls with the hot vegetables and stock, garnished with extra mint. If you prefer a thicker sauce, drain the stock into a small saucepan and boil rapidly to reduce by half.

tarragon chicken with mushrooms

low-calorie cooking oil spray

4 skinless chicken legs, 1.2 kg
(2 lb 6 oz) in total

2 leeks, sliced

175 g (6 oz) closed-cap
mushrooms, sliced

1 tablespoon plain flour

1 teaspoon mustard powder

450 ml (¾ pint) chicken stock

2 tablespoons chopped
tarragon, plus extra to garnish

3 tablespoons sherry (optional)

125 g (4 oz) fine green beans

salt and pepper

1 Preheat the slow cooker if necessary. Spray a large frying pan with a little low-calorie cooking oil spray and place over a high heat until hot. Add the chicken legs and cook for 4–5 minutes, turning once, until golden. Transfer to the slow cooker pot.

2 Add a little extra low-calorie cooking oil spray to the pan if necessary, then add the white leek slices (reserving the green slices) and the mushrooms and cook for 2–3 minutes. Stir in the flour, then add the mustard powder, stock, tarragon and sherry, if using. Season to taste and bring to the boil, stirring.

3 Pour the liquid and vegetables over the chicken, cover and cook on Low for 8–9 hours until the chicken is tender and cooked through.

4 Stir the casserole, then add the remaining green leek slices and the green beans. Cover again and cook on High for 15–30 minutes until the vegetables are tender. Spoon into shallow bowls and serve garnished with a little extra tarragon.

---

for garlicky mash, to serve as an accompaniment

CALORIES PER SERVING 122

Peel and cut 625 g (1¼ lb) potatoes into chunks and cook in a saucepan of lightly salted boiling water for about 15 minutes until tender. Drain and mash with 3 tablespoons chicken stock, 2 crushed garlic cloves and a little salt and pepper.

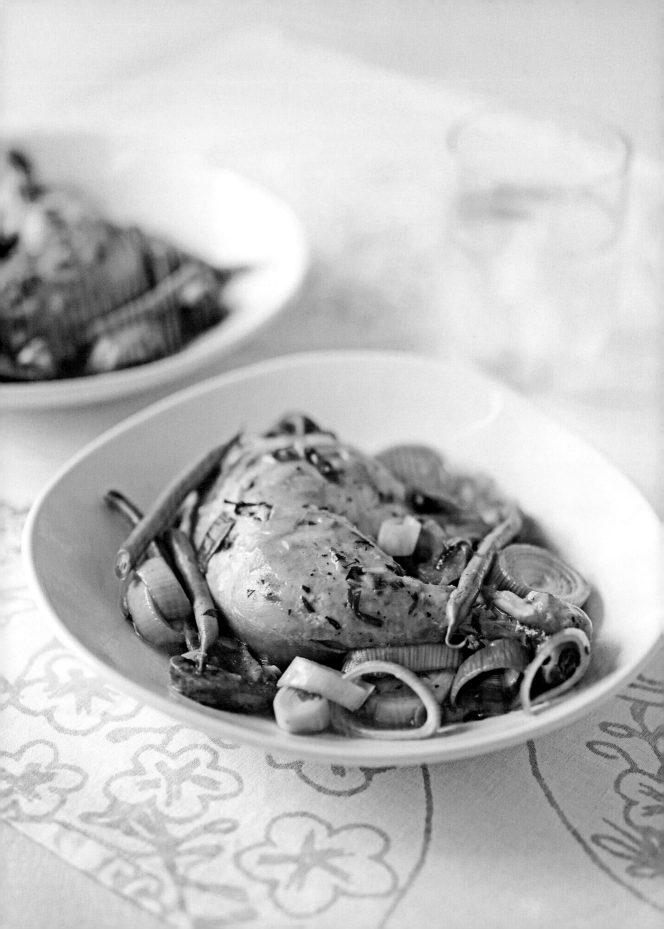

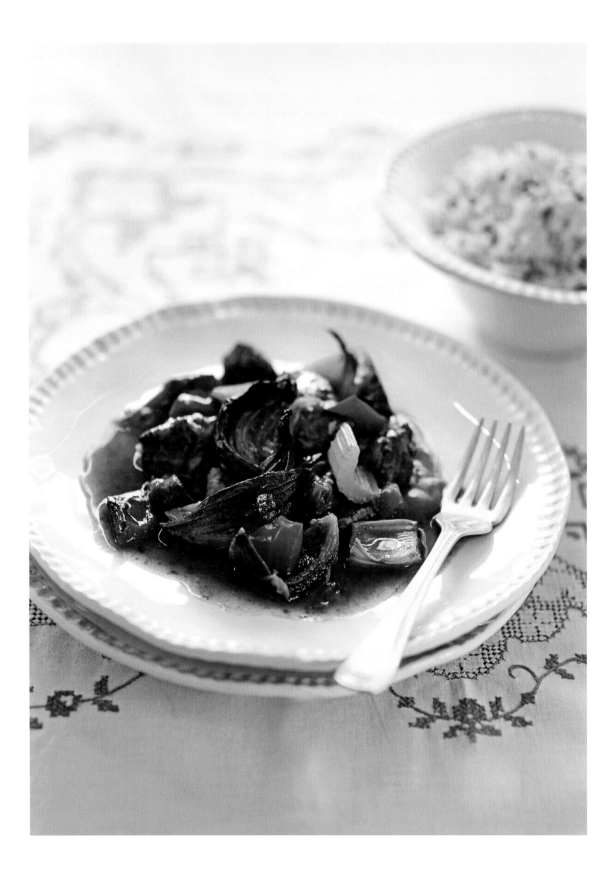

spiced beef & red pepper stew

low-calorie cooking oil spray

500 g (1 lb) stewing beef,
   trimmed of fat and cubed

2 red onions, cut into wedges

2 celery sticks, thickly sliced

2 red peppers, cored,
   deseeded and cut into chunks

2 garlic cloves, finely chopped

1 teaspoon cumin seeds,
   roughly crushed

1 teaspoon chilli powder

2 teaspoons plain flour

450 ml (¾ pint) beef stock

1 tablespoon tomato purée

salt and pepper

TO SERVE

4 tablespoons chopped fresh
   coriander

250 g (8 oz) long-grain rice,
   boiled

1   Preheat the slow cooker if necessary. Spray a large frying pan with a little low-calorie cooking oil spray and place over a high heat until hot. Add the beef, a few pieces at a time until all the beef is in the pan, and cook for 5 minutes, stirring, until browned. Use a slotted spoon to transfer the beef to the slow cooker pot.

2   Add a little more low-calorie cooking oil spray to the pan, add the onion wedges and cook for 2–3 minutes, stirring. Add the celery and red pepper, then stir in the garlic, cumin and chilli powder and cook for 1 minute.

3   Stir in the flour, then add the stock and tomato purée, season to taste and bring to the boil, stirring. Spoon over the beef, cover and cook on Low for 8–10 hours until the beef is tender.

4   Stir the chopped coriander into the cooked rice and spoon into shallow bowls. Stir the beef casserole, spoon over the rice and serve.

---

for gingered beef & noodles

CALORIES PER SERVING 490

Follow the recipe above, replacing the cumin seeds and chilli powder with 2 tablespoons soy sauce and 2 tablespoons finely chopped fresh root ginger. Serve with 250 g (8 oz) egg noodles, cooked according to packet instructions.

---

pulled pork

700 g (1 lb 6 oz) boneless pork
  shoulder joint, trimmed of fat
1 tablespoon treacle
½ teaspoon ground allspice
½ teaspoon ground ginger
½ teaspoon ground cumin
½ teaspoon dried chilli flakes
¼ teaspoon salt
leaves from 2–3 thyme sprigs
1 onion, sliced
200 ml (7 fl oz) hot chicken
  stock
pepper

TO SERVE
4 hamburger buns, split
4 lettuce leaves, shredded
3 tomatoes, thinly sliced
1 dill cucumber, drained and
  sliced

1 Preheat the slow cooker if necessary. Unroll the pork joint and make a cut through the middle to reduce the thickness by half. Place in the slow cooker pot and spread with the treacle.

2 Mix the ground spices, chilli flakes, salt and thyme leaves and season with pepper. Rub over the pork joint, then tuck the onion slices around it. Pour the hot stock over the onions, then cover and cook on High for 5–6 hours or until the pork is very tender.

3 Place the pork on a chopping board and pull into shreds using two forks. Top the bottom halves of the buns with the lettuce, tomato and dill cucumber, then pile the hot pork on top. Add a few of the onion slices to each bun and drizzle with the cooking juices. Replace the tops of the buns and serve immediately.

---

for herby pulled pork
CALORIES PER SERVING 408

Follow the recipe above to prepare the pork and spread it with the treacle. Mix the chilli flakes, salt and thyme leaves with 2 finely chopped sage sprigs and rub over the treacle-spread pork. Add the onion and stock and continue as above.

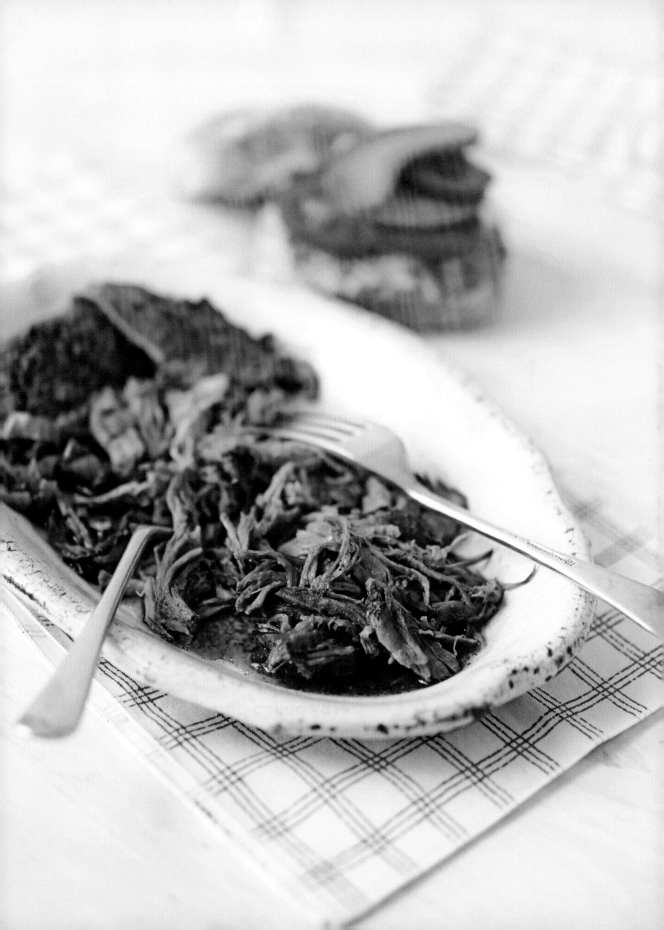

tuna arrabiata

1 tablespoon olive oil

1 onion, chopped

2 garlic cloves, finely chopped

1 red pepper, cored, deseeded and diced

1 teaspoon smoked paprika

¼–½ teaspoon dried chilli flakes

400 g (13 oz) can chopped tomatoes

150 ml (¼ pint) vegetable or fish stock

200 g (7 oz) can tuna in water, drained

salt and pepper

TO SERVE

375 g (12 oz) dried spaghetti

4 tablespoons grated Parmesan cheese

small handful of basil leaves

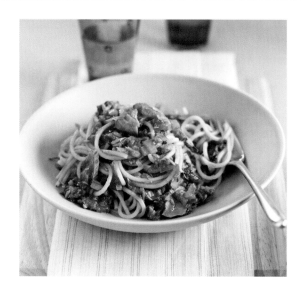

for double tomato arrabiata

CALORIES PER SERVING 479

Follow the recipe above using 75 g (3 oz) sliced sun-dried tomatoes and 100 g (3½ oz) sliced button mushrooms instead of the tuna. Cook and serve as above.

1 Preheat the slow cooker if necessary. Heat the oil in a large frying pan over a medium heat, add the onion and cook, stirring, for 5 minutes or until just browning around the edges. Add the garlic, red pepper, paprika and dried chillies and cook for 2 minutes.

2 Add the tomatoes and stock and season to taste. Bring to the boil, then transfer to the slow cooker pot. Break the tuna into large pieces and stir into the tomato mixture. Cover and cook on Low for 4-5 hours.

3 Meanwhile, cook the spaghetti in a saucepan of lightly salted boiling water according to packet instructions until tender. Drain and stir into the tomato sauce. Spoon into shallow bowls and sprinkle with the grated Parmesan and basil leaves.

tipsy mustard pork

low-calorie cooking oil spray

4 pork loin chops on the bone, 225 g (7½ oz) each, trimmed of fat

1 onion, chopped

1 tablespoon plain flour

2 teaspoons wholegrain mustard

1 teaspoon ground turmeric

150 ml (¼ pint) dry cider

300 ml (½ pint) chicken stock

500 g (1 lb) swede, cut into 2.5 cm (1 inch) pieces

250 g (8 oz) potatoes, cut into 2.5 cm (1 inch) pieces

1 dessert apple, cored and thickly sliced

salt and pepper

200 g (7 oz) sugar snap peas, steamed, to serve

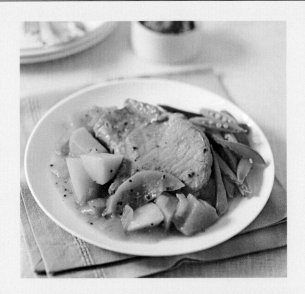

for mustard chicken with celeriac

CALORIES PER SERVING 413

Follow the recipe above, browning 4 skinless chicken leg joints in the frying pan instead of the pork chops. Continue, replacing the swede with 500 g (1 lb) diced celeriac. Cook on Low for 8–10 hours until the chicken is cooked through with no hint of pink juices and the celeriac is tender.

1   Preheat the slow cooker if necessary. Spray a large frying pan with a little low-calorie cooking oil spray and place over a high heat until hot. Add the chops in a single layer, cook for 5 minutes, turning once, until browned on both sides, then transfer to a plate.

2   Add a little extra low-calorie cooking oil spray to the pan if necessary, then add the onion and cook over a medium heat for 4–5 minutes until softened. Stir in the flour, then add the mustard, turmeric, cider and stock. Season to taste and bring to the boil, stirring.

3   Place the swede and potato in the slow cooker pot. Arrange the pork chops in a single layer on top, then add the apple slices. Pour over the hot stock mixture, cover and cook on High for 4–5 hours until the pork is very tender.

4   Transfer the pork to a plate. Divide the vegetables between 4 shallow dishes, top with the chops and drizzle with the sauce. Serve with steamed sugar snap peas.

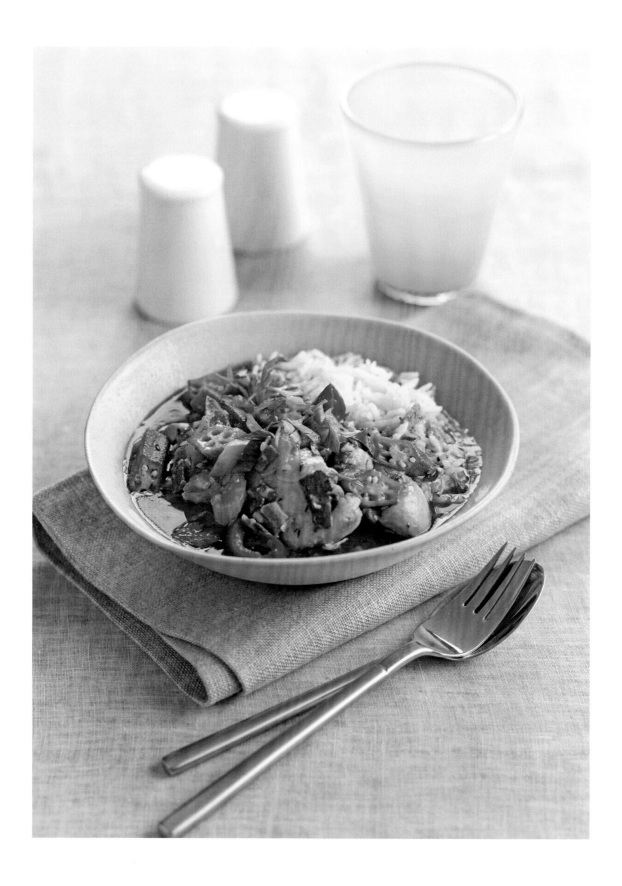

chicken gumbo

2 tablespoons olive oil

500 g (1 lb) boneless, skinless
 chicken thighs, cubed

75 g (3 oz) chorizo, diced

75 g (3 oz) smoked bacon,
 trimmed of fat and diced

1 onion, sliced

2 garlic cloves, chopped

2 tablespoons plain flour

600 ml (1 pint) chicken stock

2 bay leaves

2 thyme sprigs

¼–½ teaspoon cayenne pepper

3 celery sticks, sliced

½ each of 3 different coloured
 peppers, cored, deseeded
 and sliced

125 g (4 oz) okra, thickly sliced
 (optional)

salt

chopped parsley, to garnish

1 Preheat the slow cooker if necessary. Heat the oil in a large frying pan over a high heat, add the chicken a few pieces at time until all the chicken is in the pan, then add the chorizo and bacon and cook for 5 minutes, stirring, until the chicken is golden. Transfer to the slow cooker pot with a slotted spoon.

2 Add the onion to the frying pan and cook over a medium heat until softened. Mix in the garlic, then stir in the flour. Gradually add the stock, stirring, then add the herbs and cayenne, to taste, and season generously. Bring to the boil, stirring.

3 Add the celery and peppers to the slow cooker pot, then pour over the hot onion mixture. Cover and cook, on Low for 8–10 hours or until the chicken is cooked through.

4 Stir in the okra, if using, cover again and cook on High for 15 minutes or until the okra has just softened. Stir once more, then sprinkle with chopped parsley. Serve with rice, if liked.

for prawn gumbo

CALORIES PER SERVING 433

Follow the recipe above omitting the chicken and replacing the chicken stock with 600 ml (1 pint) fish stock, and adding 2 sliced carrots, 2 diced sweet potatoes and 1 diced courgette to the slow cooker pot with the celery and peppers. Add 200 g (7 oz) large cooked peeled prawns to the pot with the okra, if using, and cook on High for 20–30 minutes or until the prawns are piping hot. Serve with rice, if liked.

GUILT-FREE TREATS

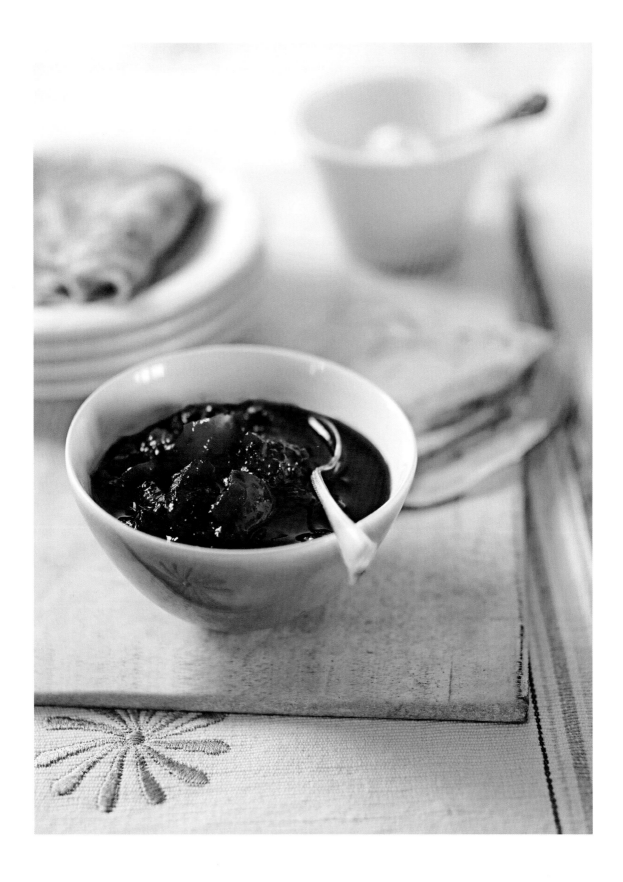

pancakes with fruit compote

300 g (10 oz) ripe red plums, halved, stoned and diced

1 dessert apple, quartered, cored and diced

150 g (5 oz) blackberries

¼ teaspoon ground cinnamon, plus extra to decorate

1 tablespoon granular sweetener

3 tablespoons water

PANCAKES

75 g (3 oz) plain flour

1 egg and 1 egg yolk

200 ml (7 fl oz) skimmed milk

1 teaspoon sunflower or vegetable oil

TO SERVE

150 g (5 oz) fromage frais

1   Preheat the slow cooker if necessary. Place all the compote ingredients in the slow cooker pot, stir well, cover and cook on High for 2–2½ hours until the fruits have softened.

2   Make the pancake batter. Place the flour in a large bowl, create a well in the middle and add the egg, egg yolk and milk. Whisk, starting from the centre and gradually drawing the flour into the eggs and milk. Once all the flour is incorporated, beat until you have a smooth, thick batter. Allow to stand for 30 minutes.

3   Heat a 7-inch frying pan over a moderate heat, wipe it with oiled kitchen paper and ladle some of the pancake batter into the pan, tilting the pan to move the batter around for a thin and even layer. Let cook for at least 30 seconds before flipping the pancake over to cook on the other side. Transfer cooked pancakes to a plate. The batter will make four 7-inch pancakes. Alternatively, use 4 ready-made pancakes, 50 g (2 oz) each.

4   Warm the pancakes and divide between 4 serving plates. Top with the fruit compote, then fold the pancakes in half and spoon the fromage frais on top. Sprinkle with a little extra cinnamon and serve immediately.

---

for orchard fruit sundaes

CALORIES PER SERVING 163

Follow the recipe above to make the fruit compote and leave to cool. Spoon into 4 glasses, top with 250 g (8 oz) fromage frais and drizzle each portion with 2 teaspoons maple syrup.

oatmeal & mixed seed granola

125 g (4 oz) medium oatmeal
50 g (2 oz) jumbo porridge
  oats
25 g (1 oz) pumpkin seeds
25 g (1 oz) sunflower seeds
15 g (½ oz) golden linseeds
¼ teaspoon ground cinnamon
1 tablespoon olive oil
3 tablespoons date syrup
juice of ½ orange
25 g (1 oz) dried goji berries

TO SERVE
600 ml (1 pint) skimmed milk
sliced banana
sliced strawberries
raspberries

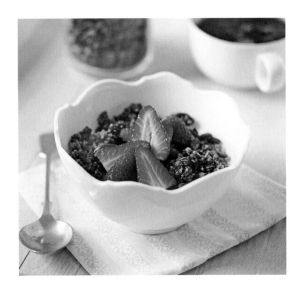

1   Preheat the slow cooker if necessary. Place the oatmeal,
    porridge oats and seeds in the slow cooker pot and stir well.
    Add the cinnamon, olive oil, date syrup and orange juice
    and mix again until thoroughly combined. Cover and cook
    on High for 1½–2 hours, stirring once or twice with a fork to
    break the mixture into clumps.

for honeyed oatmeal & fruit granola

CALORIES PER SERVING 431

Follow the recipe above,
omitting the pumpkin seeds
and using 3 tablespoons runny
honey instead of the date syrup.
Add 25 g (1 oz) dried cranberries
and 25 g (1 oz) dried cherries
instead of the goji berries and
serve as above.

2   Remove the lid and cook for 1 hour more until the granola is
    crisp. Break up once more with a fork, add the goji berries,
    then leave to cool. Store in an airtight jar in the refrigerator
    until ready to serve.

3   Serve in bowls, topped with skimmed milk and the fruit.

vanilla breakfast prunes & figs

1 breakfast tea teabag
600 ml (1 pint) boiling water
150 g (5 oz) pitted prunes
150 g (5 oz) dried figs
75 g (3 oz) caster sugar
1 teaspoon vanilla extract
pared rind of ½ orange

TO SERVE
natural yogurt
muesli

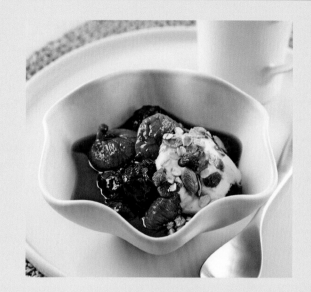

1   Preheat the slow cooker if necessary. Put the teabag into a jug or teapot, add the boiling water and leave to soak for 2–3 minutes. Remove the teabag and pour the tea into the slow cooker pot.

2   Add the whole prunes and figs, the sugar and vanilla extract to the hot tea, sprinkle with the orange rind and mix together. Cover with the lid and cook on low for 8–10 hours or overnight.

3   Serve hot with spoonfuls of natural yogurt and a sprinkling of muesli.

for breakfast apricots in orange
CALORIES PER SERVING 295

Put 300 g (10 oz) dried apricots, 50 g (2 oz) caster sugar, 300 ml (½ pint) boiling water and 150 ml (¼ pint) orange juice in the slow cooker pot. Cover and cook as above.

pineapple upside-down puddings

4 tablespoons golden syrup

2 tablespoons light muscovado sugar

220 g (7½ oz) can pineapple chunks, drained

40 g (1½ oz) glacé cherries, roughly chopped

50 g (2 oz) sunflower margarine, plus extra for greasing

50 g (2 oz) caster sugar

50 g (2 oz) self-raising flour

25 g (1 oz) desiccated coconut

1 egg

1 tablespoon milk

1 Preheat the slow cooker if necessary. Lightly grease 4 metal pudding basins, 250 ml (8 fl oz) each, and line the bases with non-stick baking paper. Divide the golden syrup and muscovado sugar between them, then place three-quarters of the pineapple on top with the cherries.

2 Place the remaining pineapple with all the remaining ingredients into a mixing bowl and beat together until smooth. Spoon the mixture into the pudding basins, level the surfaces with the back of a small spoon, then cover the tops with greased foil and put in the slow cooker pot.

3 Pour boiling water into the slow cooker pot to come halfway up the sides of the basins, cover and cook on High for 2–2½ hours until the sponge is well risen and springs back when pressed with a fingertip. Remove the foil, loosen the edges of the puddings with a round-bladed knife and turn out into shallow bowls. Peel away the lining paper and serve.

---

for plum & almond puddings

CALORIES PER SERVING 393

Follow the recipe above, using 4 stoned and sliced red plums instead of the pineapple and cherries. Omit the coconut and add 25 g (1 oz) ground almonds and a few drops of almond essence to the sponge mixture instead.

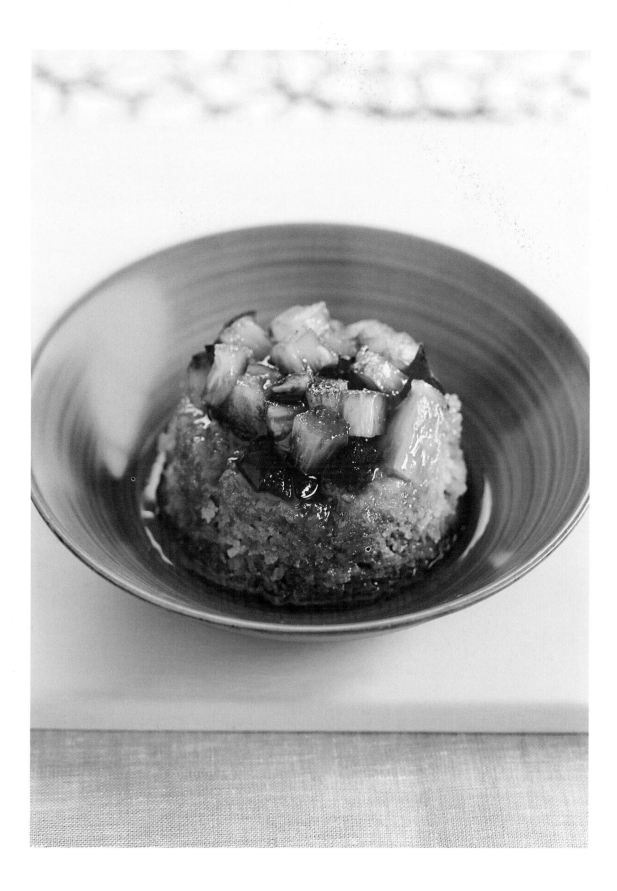

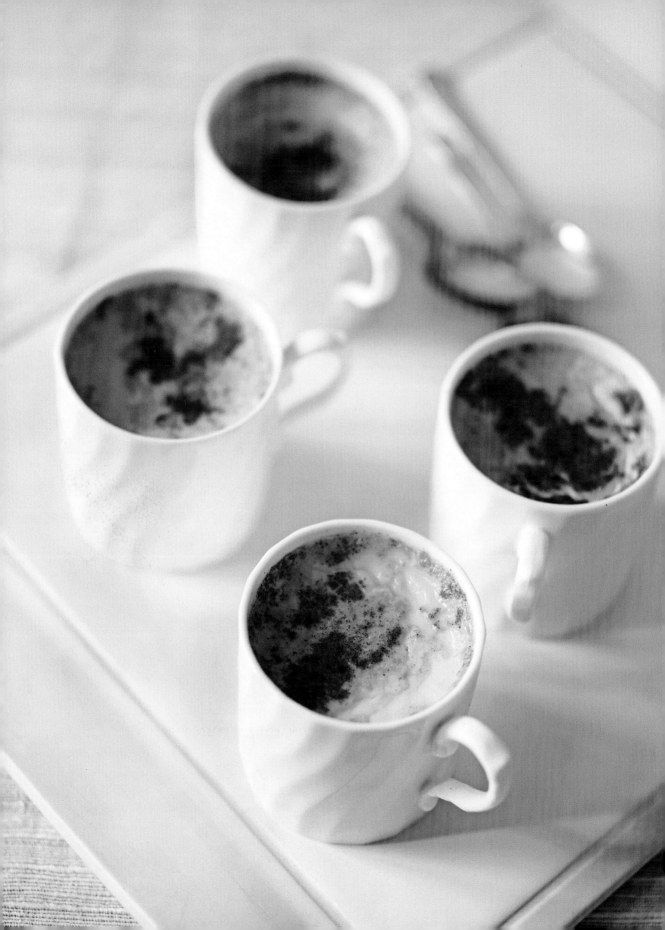

baked honey & orange custards

2 eggs

2 egg yolks

400 ml (14 fl oz) semi skimmed
  milk

3 teaspoons granular
  sweetener

3 teaspoons runny honey

½ teaspoon vanilla extract

finely grated rind of orange,
  plus extra to garnish

large pinch of ground
  cinnamon

1 Preheat the slow cooker if necessary. Place the eggs, egg
yolks and milk in a mixing bowl with the sweetener, honey and
vanilla and whisk together until smooth. Strain the mixture
through a sieve into a large jug, then whisk in the orange rind.

2 Divide the mixture between 4 x 150 ml (¼ pint) ovenproof
dishes (checking first that the dishes fit in your slow cooker
pot). Place the dishes in the slow cooker pot and sprinkle the
cinnamon over the top. Pour hot water into the slow cooker
pot until it comes halfway up the sides of the dishes. Cover
the tops of the dishes with foil, place the lid on the slow
cooker and cook on Low for 4–5 hours until set.

3 Remove the dishes from the slow cooker and leave to cool.
Transfer to the refrigerator to chill well before serving,
garnished with a little extra orange rind.

---

for vanilla crème brulée

CALORIES PER SERVING 193

Follow the recipe above to cook and chill the custards, using
1 teaspoon vanilla extract and omitting the orange rind and
cinnamon. Just before serving, sprinkle 1 teaspoon caster
sugar over the top of each dish and caramelize the sugar with a
cook's blow torch or under a preheated hot grill. Cool for a few
minutes to allow the sugar to set hard, then serve with a few
fresh raspberries.

coconut & rose rice pudding

65 g (2½ oz) pudding rice,
   rinsed in cold water and
   drained
50 g (2 oz) caster sugar
25 g (1 oz) desiccated coconut
600 ml (1 pint) semi skimmed
   milk
½-1 teaspoon rose water,
   to taste

TO SERVE
125 g (4 oz) raspberries
2 teaspoons desiccated
   coconut

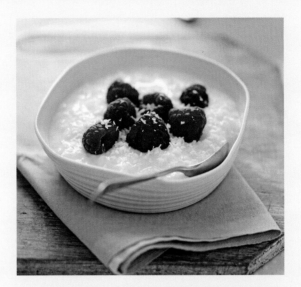

1   Preheat the slow cooker if necessary. Place the rice, sugar
    and coconut in the slow cooker pot, add the milk and stir
    well. Cover and cook on High for 2½-3 hours until the
    rice is tender.

for vanilla & orange rice pudding

CALORIES PER SERVING 233

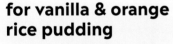

Split 1 vanilla pod lengthways
and scrape out the seeds with
a small knife. Follow the recipe
above, adding the vanilla seeds
to the rice and milk in the slow
cooker pot with the vanilla pod
and the finely grated rind of
½ orange. Stir well, cover and
cook as above. Stir again and
remove the vanilla pod before
serving with raspberries and a
sprinkling of coconut.

2   Stir well, then add the rose water, to taste. Spoon into bowls,
    top with the raspberries and a little extra coconut and
    serve immediately.

brandied chocolate fondue

100 g (3½ oz) dark chocolate,
  broken into pieces
6 tablespoons skimmed milk
1 teaspoon granular sweetener
1 tablespoon brandy

TO SERVE
500 g (1 lb) strawberries,
  halved if large
150 g (5 oz) raspberries
1 large peach, halved, stoned
  and cut into chunks

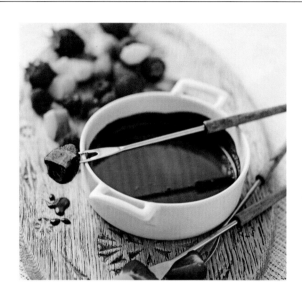

1   Preheat the slow cooker if necessary. Place the chocolate, milk
    and sweetener in a heatproof bowl, cover with a saucer and
    stand in the slow cooker pot. Pour boiling water into the slow
    cooker pot to come halfway up the sides of the bowl, cover
    and cook on High for ¾–1 hour.

2   Remove the bowl from the slow cooker and stand on a large
    plate. Stir the fondue until smooth and glossy, then stir in
    the brandy.

3   Arrange the strawberries, raspberries and peaches on the
    plate. Serve with fondue forks or wooden skewers for spearing
    the fruit and dipping into the fondue.

for white chocolate fondue

CALORIES PER SERVING 213

Place 100 g (3½ oz) white
chocolate, broken into pieces,
in a heatproof bowl with a few
drops of vanilla extract and
6 tablespoons skimmed milk.
Cook as above, then stir in
1 tablespoon Kirsch and serve
with mixed berries.

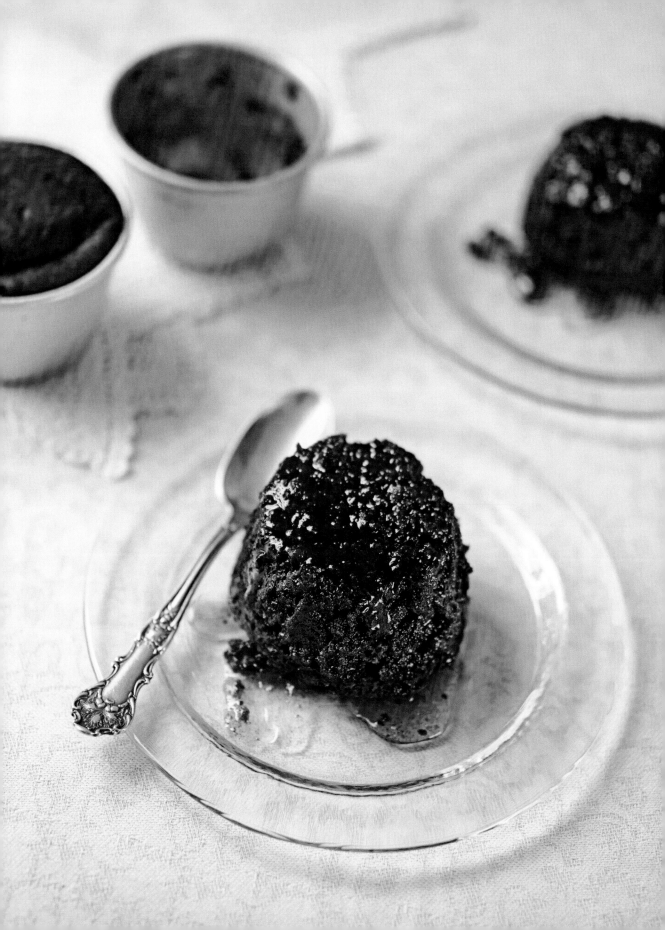

gingered date & syrup puddings

125 g (4 oz) pitted dates, chopped

125 ml (4 fl oz) boiling water

¼ teaspoon bicarbonate of soda

50 g (2 oz) sunflower margarine, plus extra for greasing

4 tablespoons golden syrup

50 g (2 oz) light muscovado sugar

100 g (3½ oz) self-raising flour

1 egg

1 teaspoon vanilla extract

1 teaspoon ground ginger

2 small scoops of low-fat vanilla ice cream

1 Preheat the slow cooker if necessary. Place the dates, boiling water and bicarbonate of soda in a bowl, stir and set aside for 10 minutes.

2 Lightly grease 4 metal pudding basins, 200 ml (7 fl oz) each, and line the bases with non-stick baking paper. Divide the golden syrup between the basins.

3 Place the margarine, sugar, flour, egg, vanilla and ginger in a food processor and blend until smooth. Drain the dates, add to the processor and blend briefly to mix. Divide the mixture between the pudding basins, cover the tops with greased foil and put in the slow cooker pot.

4 Pour boiling water into the slow cooker pot to come halfway up the sides of the basins, cover and cook on High for 3½–4 hours until the sponge is well risen and springs back when pressed with a fingertip.

5 Remove the foil, loosen the edges of the puddings with a round-bladed knife and turn out into shallow bowls. Peel away the lining paper and serve immediately with the ice cream.

---

for sticky banana puddings

CALORIES PER SERVING 411

Omit the dates, boiling water and bicarbonate of soda. Follow the recipe above, adding 1 ripe banana to the food processor with the remaining ingredients. Blend and continue as above.

plum & blueberry swirl

300 g (10 oz) ripe red plums,
   halved, stoned and cut into
   chunks
150 g (5 oz) blueberries
1 tablespoon granular
   sweetener
juice of ½ orange
3 tablespoons water
1 tablespoon cornflour

YOGURT
200 g (7 oz) 0% fat Greek
   yogurt
finely grated rind of ½ orange
1 tablespoon granular
   sweetener

for minted strawberry & blueberry swirl
CALORIES PER SERVING 102

Place 300 g (10 oz) ripe
strawberries in the slow cooker
pot with 150 g (5 oz) blueberries,
1 tablespoon sweetener and the
juice of ½ orange. Cook as above,
then thicken with the cornflour,
cook for a further 15 minutes and
leave to cool. Mix 200 g
(7 oz) 0% fat Greek yogurt with
1 tablespoon chopped mint and
1 tablespoon granular sweetener,
then swirl with the fruit as above.

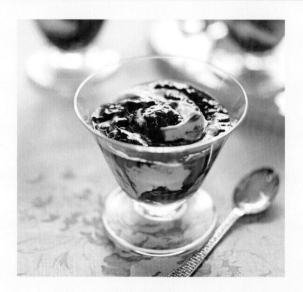

1 Preheat the slow cooker if necessary. Place the plums
and blueberries in the slow cooker pot, sprinkle with the
sweetener, then add the orange juice and water. Cover and
cook on High for 2–2½ hours until the fruit is soft.

2 Mix the cornflour to a smooth paste with a little cold water
and stir into the pot. Cover again and cook for a further
15 minutes until thickened, stir the fruit and leave to cool.

3 Mix the yogurt with the orange rind and sweetener. Divide
the fruit between 4 serving glasses, top with the yogurt,
then swirl together with a teaspoon. Chill until ready
to serve.

spiced pears

300 ml (½ pint) hot water

4 cardamom pods, crushed

7.5 cm (3 inch) cinnamon stick, halved

2.5 cm (1 inch) piece of fresh root ginger, thinly sliced

2 teaspoons granular sweetener

4 pears with stalks, peeled, halved lengthways and cored

pared rind and juice of 1 lemon

pared rind and juice of 1 orange

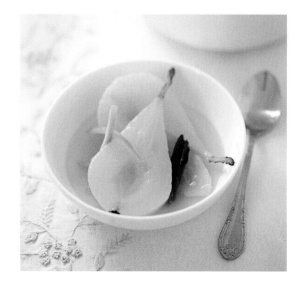

1 Preheat the slow cooker if necessary. Pour the hot water into the slow cooker pot, then stir in the cardamom pods and their black seeds, the cinnamon, ginger and sweetener.

2 Add the pears and the lemon and orange juice, then gently turn the pears in the liquid to coat and arrange them cut sides down in a single layer. Cut the pared lemon and orange rind into very thin strips and sprinkle on top.

3 Cover and cook on Low for 3–4 hours until the pears are tender. The cooking time will depend on their ripeness. Serve warm.

for mulled wine pears

CALORIES PER SERVING 99

Follow the recipe above, using 150 ml (¼ pint) red wine and 150 ml (¼ pint) hot water instead of 300 ml (½ pint) hot water, and using 4 cloves instead of the cardamom pods. Increase the sweetener to 3 teaspoons, or to taste, and cook as above.

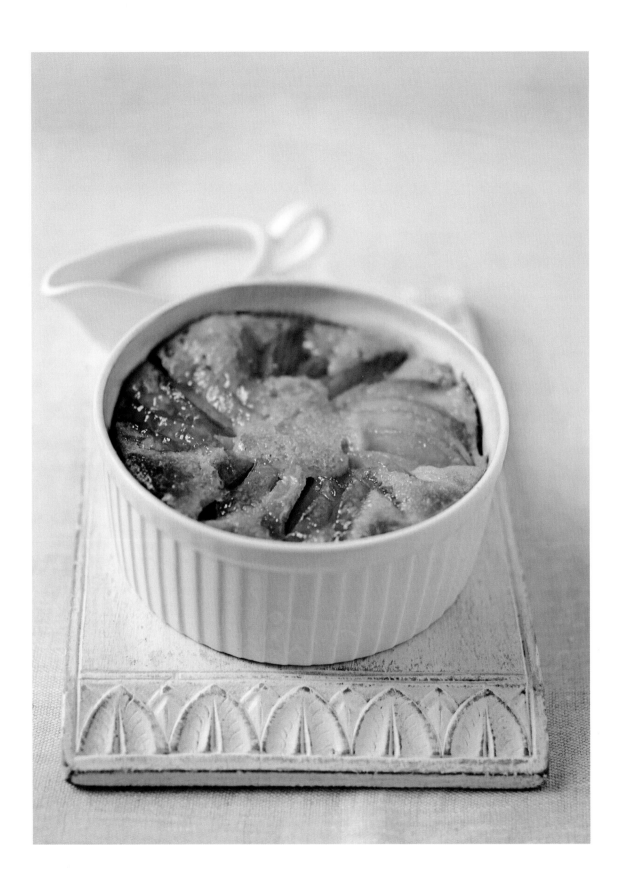

eve's pudding

50 g (2 oz) sunflower margarine, plus extra for greasing

50 g (2 oz) caster sugar

50 g (2 oz) self-raising flour

25 g (1 oz) ground almonds

¼ teaspoon baking powder

1 egg

grated rind and juice of 1 lemon

1 dessert apple, quartered, cored and sliced

1 tablespoon apricot jam

75 g (3 oz) instant powdered custard with sweetener, to serve

1 Preheat the slow cooker if necessary. Grease the base and sides of a 15 cm (6 inch) round ovenproof dish, about 6 cm (2½ inches) deep, with a little margarine. Place the margarine, sugar, flour, almonds and baking powder in a food processor, add the egg and lemon rind and blend until smooth. Spoon into the dish and spread level.

2 Toss the apple slices with the lemon juice, then overlap in a ring on top of the pudding mixture. Cover the dish with greased foil and put in the slow cooker pot. Pour boiling water into the slow cooker pot to come halfway up the sides of the dish, cover and cook on High for 3–3½ hours until a knife comes out cleanly when inserted into the centre.

3 Dot the top of the pudding with the apricot jam, then gently spread into an even layer. Place under a preheated hot grill for 3–4 minutes until the top is lightly caramelized. Make the custard with boiling water according to packet instructions and serve with the pudding.

for chocolate & pear pudding

CALORIES PER SERVING 265

Follow the recipe above to make the pudding base, using 1 tablespoon cocoa powder instead of the lemon rind. Quarter, core and slice 1 small pear, toss with the lemon juice, then arrange over the pudding mixture. Cover and bake as above, then dust the top with a little sifted icing sugar before serving.

baked apples with blackberries

4 Gala dessert apples, 425 g
   (14 oz) in total
150 g (5 oz) blackberries
1 tablespoon blackberry or
   blueberry jam
6 tablespoons pressed
   apple juice

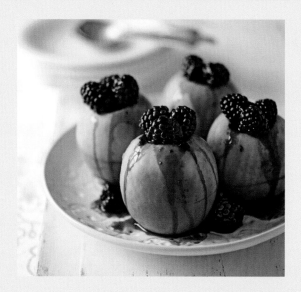

1 Preheat the slow cooker if necessary. Use an apple corer
   or small knife to remove the cores from the apples, then
   enlarge the holes slightly at the top and place the apples in
   the slow cooker pot.

2 Press a few of the blackberries into the apple cavities, then
   dot with jam. Push the remaining berries into the cavities,
   then pour the apple juice into the slow cooker pot. Cover
   and cook on High for 3–3 ½ hours until the apples are soft
   but still a bright colour.

3 Serve in shallow bowls with some of the juice spooned over.

for christmas baked apples

CALORIES PER SERVING 119

Core the apples as above and
place in the slow cooker pot.
Mix 4 teaspoons Christmas
mincemeat with a large pinch of
ground cinnamon and 40 g
(1 ½ oz) diced ready-to-eat dried
apricots. Use the mixture to fill
the apples, pour 6 tablespoons
apple juice into the slow cooker
pot and cook as above.

apricot & cardamom fool

325 g (11 oz) apricots,
   halved, stoned and cut into
   chunks
2 cardamom pods, crushed
1 tablespoon runny honey
4 tablespoons water
150 g (5 oz) ready-made
   custard
150 g (5 oz) fromage frais

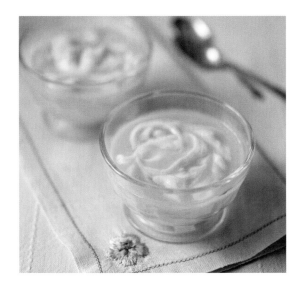

1   Preheat the slow cooker if necessary. Place the apricots in
    the slow cooker pot with the crushed cardamom pods and
    their black seeds. Drizzle over the honey and water, cover
    and cook on Low for 1½–2 hours until the apricots are soft.

2   Remove the pot from the slow cooker and leave to cool for
    30 minutes. Discard the cardamom pods and purée the
    fruit in a liquidizer or with a hand-held stick blender.

for plum &
cinnamon fool

CALORIES PER SERVING 131

Place 325 g (11 oz) chopped ripe
red plums in the slow cooker
pot with ½ teaspoon ground
cinnamon, 1 tablespoon runny
honey and 4 tablespoons
water. Cook as above, allow to
cool, then purée. Swirl with the
custard and fromage frais, chill
and serve as for the main recipe.

3   Mix the custard with the fromage frais and place a spoonful
    in each of 4 serving glasses. Add a spoonful of the fruit
    mixture and continue alternating custard and fruit to fill the
    glasses. Swirl the ingredients together with the handle of a
    teaspoon and chill until ready to serve.

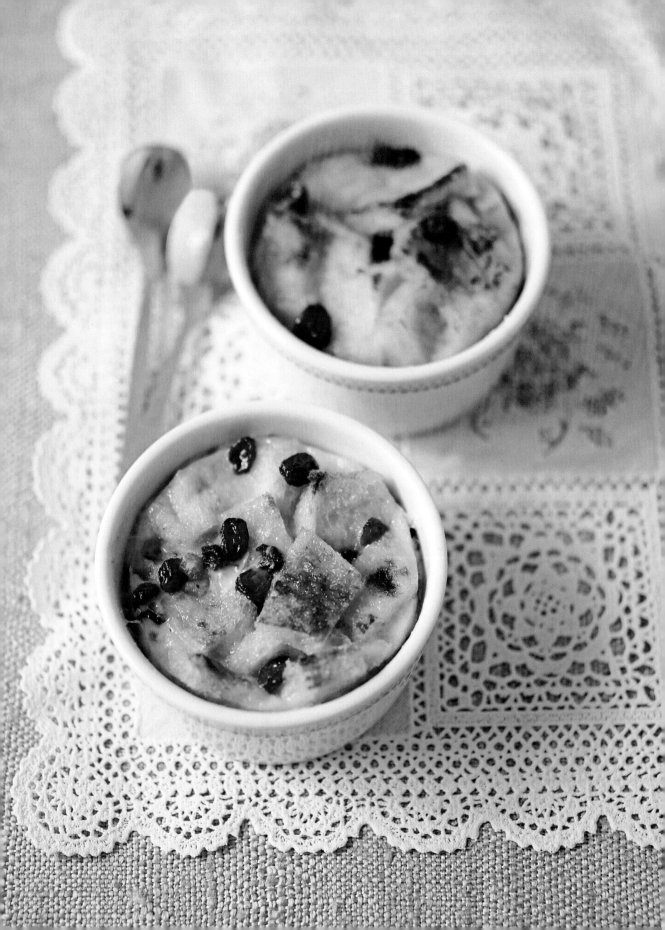

sherried bread & butter puddings

50 g (2 oz) mixed dried fruit

2 tablespoons sweet or
dry sherry

1 tablespoon sunflower
margarine

100 g (3½ oz) white bread
slices

6 teaspoons caster sugar

200 ml (7 fl oz) skimmed milk

1 teaspoon vanilla extract

2 eggs

1 Preheat the slow cooker if necessary. Place the dried fruit and sherry in a small saucepan and bring just to the boil. Remove from the heat and set aside.

2 Grease 4 x 200 ml (7 fl oz) heatproof dishes with a little margarine, then use the rest to spread on the bread. Cut the bread into cubes, then layer in the dishes with the sherried fruit and 4 teaspoons of the sugar.

3 Beat the milk, vanilla and eggs in a jug, then strain into the dishes. Cover with squares of greased foil and stand in the slow cooker pot. Pour hot water into the pot to come halfway up the sides of the dishes, then cover and cook on Low for 3½–4 hours or until the custard has set.

4 Sprinkle the tops of the puddings with the remaining sugar and brown with a cook's blow torch, or under a preheated hot grill. Serve warm.

---

for paddington puddings
CALORIES PER SERVING 214

Spread 100 g (3½ oz) white bread slices with 1 tablespoon sunflower margarine and 2 tablespoons reduced-sugar fine-shred marmalade. Layer in the dishes with 50 g (2 oz) dried fruit. Mix the milk, vanilla and eggs, as above, with 2 teaspoons caster sugar and pour over the bread mixture. Cook and finish as above.

chocolate crème caramels

2 tablespoons cocoa powder

2 teaspoons instant coffee

2 tablespoons boiling water

2 eggs

2 egg yolks

2 tablespoons granular
   sweetener

450 ml (¾ pint) semi skimmed
   milk

CARAMEL

100 g (3½ oz) granulated sugar

6 tablespoons cold water

2 tablespoons boiling water

1 Preheat the slow cooker if necessary. For the caramel, place the granulated sugar in a heavy-based saucepan with the cold water. Cook over a low heat, without stirring, until the sugar has completely dissolved. Increase the heat and boil for 5-8 minutes or until the syrup turns a rich golden brown, but before it becomes too dark.

2 Remove the pan from the heat and add the boiling water, taking care as the syrup can spit. Tilt the pan to mix, then pour into 4 x 200 ml (7 fl oz) metal pudding basins. Holding the basins with a cloth, tilt them to swirl the caramel over the base and sides. Cool for 10 minutes.

3 Place the cocoa, coffee and boiling water in a mixing bowl and stir to a smooth paste. Add the eggs, egg yolks and sweetener and stir until smooth.

4 Pour the milk into the empty caramel pan and bring just to the boil. Gradually whisk it into the cocoa mixture, then strain through a sieve into a jug. Pour into the basins, cover the tops with greased foil and put in the slow cooker pot.

5 Pour boiling water into the slow cooker pot to come halfway up the sides of the basins, cover and cook on Low for 3-4 hours until set. Remove from the slow cooker and leave to cool, then chill in the refrigerator for 3-4 hours or overnight. To serve, dip the moulds in hot water, count to 10, loosen the edges with a round-bladed knife, then turn out onto shallow dishes.

for vanilla crème caramels

CALORIES PER SERVING 239

Follow the recipe above to make the caramel and put it in the basins. Mix 2 eggs with 3 egg yolks, 2 tablespoons granular sweetener and 1 teaspoon vanilla extract. Add the hot milk and continue as above.

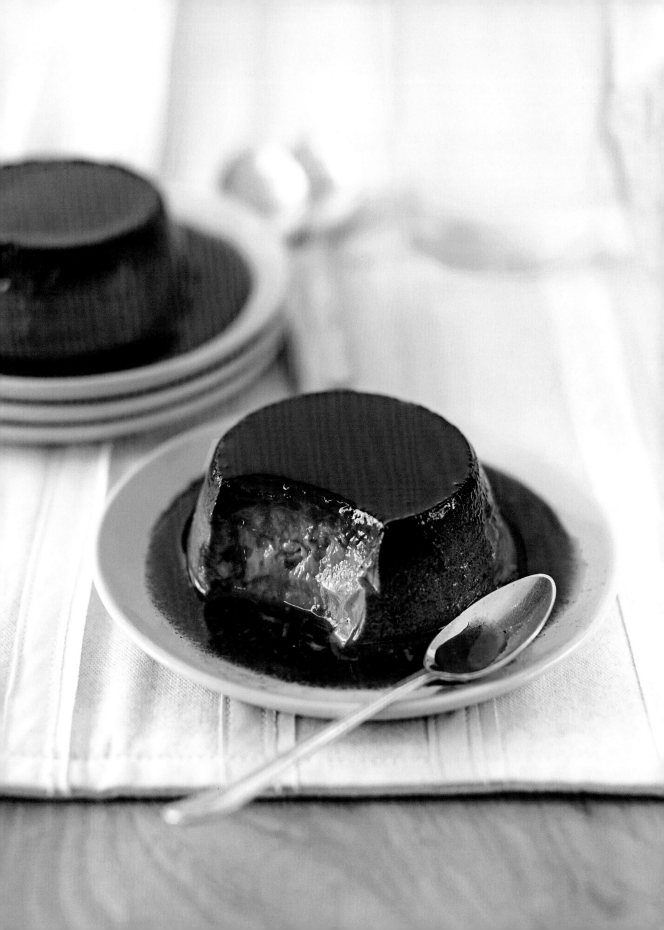

honeyed rice pudding

butter, for greasing
750 ml (1¼ pints) full-fat
  Jersey milk
3 tablespoons set honey
125 g (4 oz) risotto rice

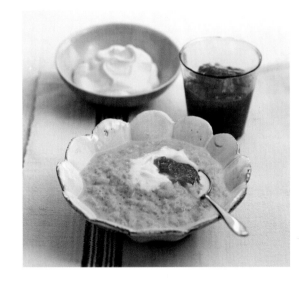

for vanilla rice pudding

CALORIES PER SERVING 364
(NOT INCLUDING CREAM)

Pour the milk into a saucepan, replace the honey with 3 tablespoons caster sugar and bring just to the boil. Slit a vanilla pod, scrape the black seeds out with a small knife and add to the milk with the pod. Pour into the greased slow cooker pot, add the rice and cook as above. Remove the vanilla pod before serving with thick cream.

1 Preheat the slow cooker if necessary; see the manufacturer's instructions. Lightly butter the inside of the slow cooker pot. Pour the milk into a saucepan, add the honey and bring just to the boil, stirring until the honey has melted. Pour into the slow cooker pot, add the rice and stir gently.

2 Cover with the lid and cook on low for 2½–3 hours, stirring once during cooking, or until the pudding is thickened and the rice is soft. Stir again just before spooning into dishes. Top each bowl with 1 tablespoon of jam and thick cream, if liked.

baked peaches with ginger

2.5 cm (1 inch) piece of fresh root ginger, finely chopped

6 ripe peaches, halved and stoned

6 tablespoons pressed apple juice

1 tablespoon caster sugar

75 g (3 oz) blueberries

150 ml (¼ pint) 0% fat Greek yogurt

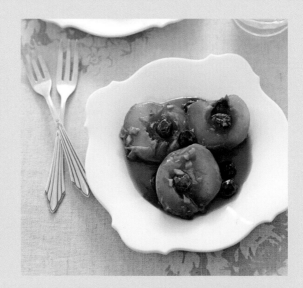

1 Preheat the slow cooker if necessary. Arrange the chopped ginger over the base of the slow cooker pot, then place the peaches, cut sides down, on top in a single layer. Pour over the apple juice, then sprinkle with the sugar and blueberries.

2 Cover and cook on Low for 1½–2½ hours until the peaches are piping hot and the juices are beginning to run from the blueberries. Spoon into serving bowls and serve warm or cold with the Greek yogurt.

for baked peaches with rosé wine

CALORIES PER SERVING 100

Arrange 8 peach halves, cut sides down, in the base of the slow cooker pot and pour over 6 tablespoons rosé wine, 1 tablespoon caster sugar and 125 g (4 oz) raspberries instead of the blueberries. Cover, cook and serve as above.

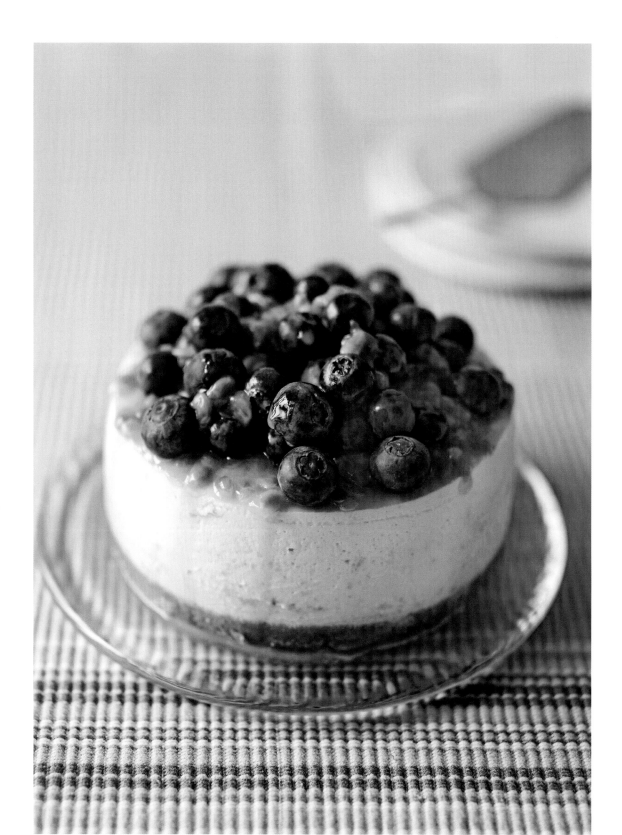

blueberry & passion fruit cheesecake

1 tablespoon sunflower margarine, plus extra for greasing

75 g (3 oz) reduced-fat digestive biscuits, finely crushed

300 g (10 oz) extra-light soft cheese

175 ml (6 fl oz) 0% fat Greek yogurt

1 tablespoon cornflour

finely grated rind and juice of ½ lime

1 teaspoon vanilla extract

3 tablespoons granular sweetener

3 tablespoons caster sugar

2 eggs

125 g (4 oz) blueberries

2 passion fruits, halved

1 Preheat the slow cooker if necessary. Grease the base and sides of a 15 cm (6 inch) round ovenproof dish, 6 cm (2½ inches) deep, with a little margarine. Line the base with non-stick baking paper.

2 Melt the margarine in a small saucepan and stir in the crushed biscuits. Spoon into the dish and press down firmly to make a thin, even layer. Place the cheese, yogurt and cornflour in a mixing bowl and whisk until smooth. Add the lime rind and juice, vanilla, sweetener, sugar and eggs and whisk again until smooth.

3 Pour the mixture into the dish and smooth the surface. Cover with greased foil and put in the slow cooker pot. Pour boiling water into the slow cooker pot to come halfway up the sides of the dish, cover and cook on High for 2–2½ hours or until the cheesecake is set but with a slight wobble in the centre. Remove from the slow cooker and leave to cool, then chill in the refrigerator for 3–4 hours or overnight.

4 Loosen the edge of the cheesecake with a knife, turn out of the dish and peel away the lining paper. Place on a serving plate, pile on the blueberries, then scoop the passion fruit seeds over them. Serve cut into wedges.

for summer berry cheesecake
CALORIES PER SERVING 345

Follow the recipe above to make the cheesecake, using the grated rind and juice of ½ lemon instead of the lime. Gently toss 100 g (3½ oz) sliced strawberries and 100 g (3½ oz) raspberries with 2 tablespoons reduced-sugar strawberry jam and 1 tablespoon lemon juice instead of the blueberries and passion fruits. Turn out the cheesecake and top with the berry mixture just before serving.

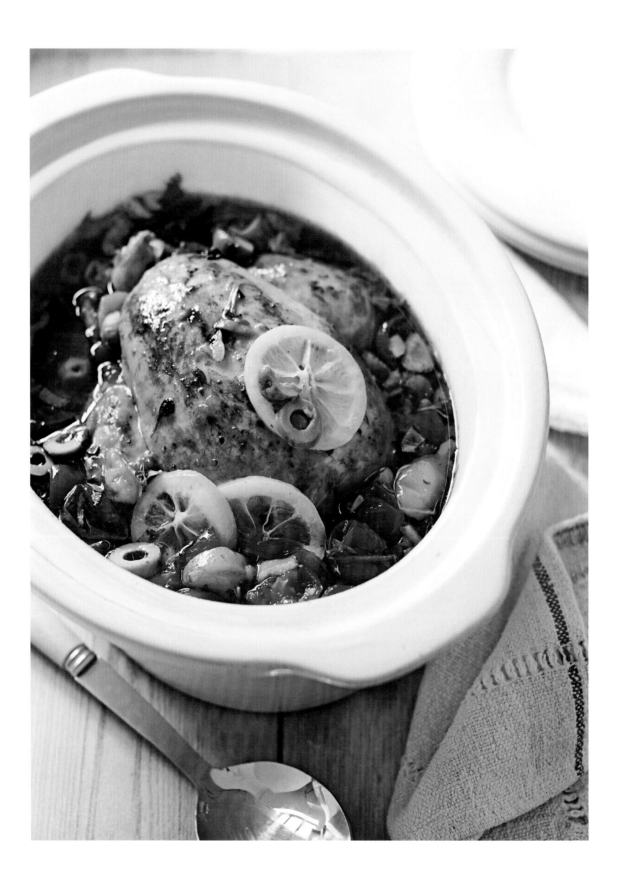

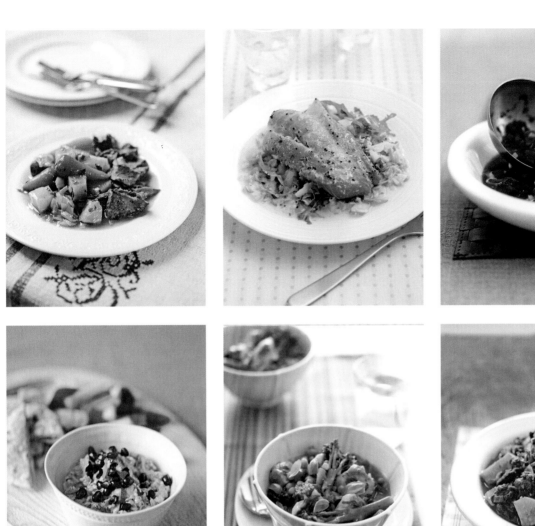

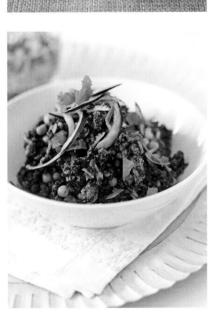

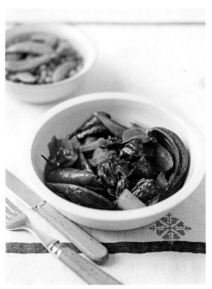

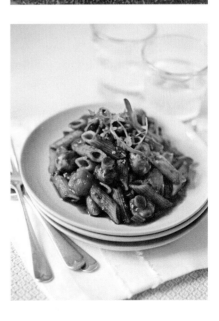

INDEX

GLOSSARY

UK	US	UK	US
aubergine	eggplant	desiccated coconut	dry unsweetened coconut
bacon rashers, back/streaky normal	bacon slices, Canadian-style	digestive biscuits	use plain cookies
		flageolet beans	great northern beans
beef, stewing	beef, chuck or round		
bicarbonate of soda	baking soda	flour, plain	flour, all-purpose
cornflour	corn-starch	flour, self-raising	use all-purpose flour plus 1 tsp baking powder per 125 g (4 oz) of flour
coriander	if referring to the leaves, cilantro		
courgette	zucchini	fromage frais	use Greek-style yogurt
creamed coconut	block of coconut meat, sold at Asian grocery store	gammon	cured ham
		golden syrup	light corn syrup

UK	US	UK	US
grill; grill rack	broil/broiler; broiler rack	puy lentils, dried	french green lentils, dried
haricot beans	navy beans	rocket	arugula
linseeds	flaxseed	single cream	light cream
mangetout	snow peas	soya mince	textured vegetable protein grounds
milk, full-fat/ semi-skinned	milk, whole/low-fat	spring onion	scallion
minced (meat)	ground	sprouting broccoli	baby broccoli (broccolini)
mixed spice	allspice	sugar, caster/icing	sugar, superfine/ confectioner's
mushrooms, chestnut	mushrooms, cremini	sultanas	golden raisins
natural yogurt	plain yogurt	swede	rutabaga
pak choi	bok choy	tomato purée	tomato paste
passata	tomato purée or sauce	treacle	molasses
prawns	shrimp	wholemeal bread	wholewheat bread
pudding basin	ovenproof bowl		
pulses, dried	beans, dried		

ACKNOWLEDGEMENTS

Publishing Director: Eleanor Maxfield
Editorial Assistant: Louisa Johnson
Art Director: Jaz Bahra
Junior Designer: Rachael Shone
Production Controller: Serena Savini

Photography copyright © Octopus Publishing Group: Stephen Conroy 2, 7, 8, 9, 10, 12, 13, 21, 22, 23, 30, 33, 34, 36, 39, 45, 59, 60, 63, 65, 71, 74, 75, 77, 82, 94, 111, 116, 124, 131, 135, 137, 150, 152, 159, 161, 178; William Shaw 16, 17, 18, 25, 27, 28, 29, 35, 42, 46, 47, 49, 51, 52, 53, 54, 57, 58, 64, 68, 73, 78, 80, 81, 85, 86, 88, 89, 90, 93, 95, 96, 98, 100, 102, 103, 105, 106, 108, 109, 112, 115, 117, 118, 121, 122, 123, 127, 128, 130, 132, 136, 139, 140, 142, 143, 145, 146, 149, 151, 156, 158, 162, 164, 165, 166, 168, 169, 170, 172, 173, 174, 177, 179, 180.

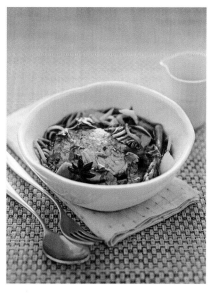
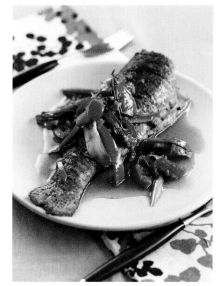
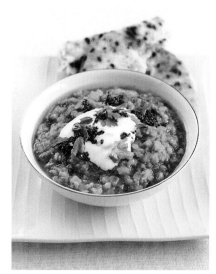
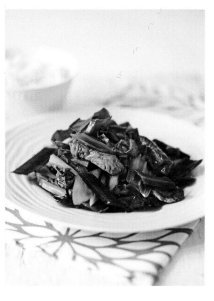
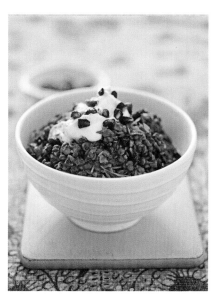
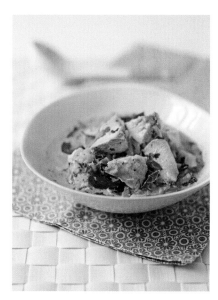
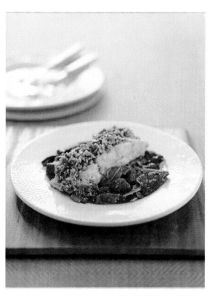
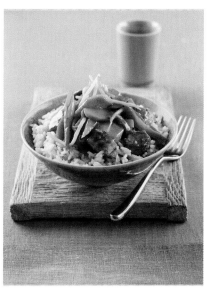
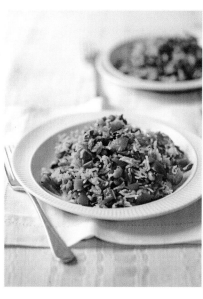

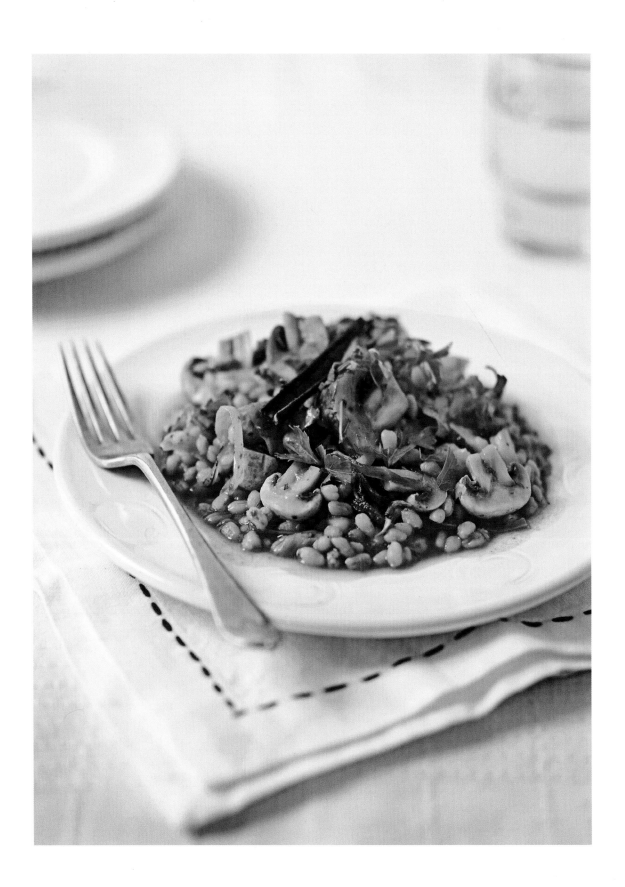